Meal by Meal

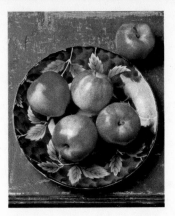

Meal *by* Meal

365 Daily Meditations for Finding Balance through Mindful Eating

DONALD ALTMAN

New World Library
Novato, California

New World Library
14 Pamaron Way
Novato, California 94949

Book design Maxine Ressler

Library of Congress Cataloging-in-Publication Data
Altman, Donald.
    Meal by meal : 365 daily meditations for finding balnce through mindful eating / Donald
Altman. – 1st ed.
       p.   cm.
ISBN 978-1-930722-30-9
1. Food—Religious aspects. 2. Spiritual life. 3. Meditations. 4. Affirmations. I. Title.

BL65.F65 A476 2004
204/.46—dc22   0406

ISBN 978-1-930722-30-9

Printed in Canada

Dedication

MAY THIS BOOK BE A BLESSING FOR ALL WHO SEEK well-being, happiness, harmony, and balance in their lives. May it be a blessing for the Earth and for all enlightened beings who bring light into the darkness.

Acknowledgments

THIS WORK IS A BLESSING WHICH HAS BEEN MADE possible through the efforts of many. My gratitude extends to all those wise beings, guides, and teachers who have helped me find a kinder, more compassionate, and enlightened way to live and work with others. In particular, I would like to thank Karen Bouris for her ongoing vision, enthusiasm, and belief in the potential of this book; editor John Nelson for his creative input, ideas, and support; disordered eating specialist Jacki Abbott for her wise guidance and sharing of experiences; Lindsey Hall for her support and thoughtfulness; Katie McMillan, Alma Bune, and the staff at Inner Ocean Publishing for all their caring effort and ideas; my agents Arielle Ford and Brian Hilliard for their guidance; friend and writer Randy Fitzgerald for his always wise and generous feedback; friend John Morley for his kind sharing of his *Wry, Wit and Wisdom* collection of quotes; my mother Barbara for always being a beacon of light and laughter; and especially, my wife Sanda for her tireless support and her nourishing meals that gave me the energy and well-being needed to create this book.

Introduction

EATING IS ONE OF OUR GREATEST JOYS. AND YET, IT CAN also be a struggle for so many. *Meal by Meal* has given me the opportunity to complete another chapter in my work to explore food's ability to bring peace and harmony into our lives. Since writing *Art of the Inner Meal: The Power of Mindful Practices to Heal Our Food Cravings*, I have worked with all sorts of people. Some had no real food concerns other than wanting to integrate the spiritual potential of food into their lives. Others had serious issues around disordered eating and wanted to find a way to manage and moderate food in their lives.

I am always humbled and amazed at how food serves as a powerful healing medium for those needing compassion and peace in their food choices and meals. The path that leads to this healing is, amazingly, an ancient one: mindfulness. While mindfulness was pioneered thousands of years ago, it is now a central component of many clinical therapy programs designed for those who need help with disordered eating and mood regulation. In my work as a mental health counselor, as well as in my Mindful Eating Workshops, I have seen mindfulness help those struggling with eating problems.

In particular, *Meal by Meal* is special because it is the first book that actually teaches mindfulness using a day-by-day, meal-by-meal approach. It can help whether you want to change unskillful eating habits, stop struggling with diets, lose your fear of food, make meals more meaningful, become less judgmental of yourself and others around the dinner table, or make food choices without second-guessing and blaming yourself afterward. For these reasons this book can benefit anyone who wants to experience and know the life-changing power of mindfulness.

What is mindfulness? Well, it is one of those elusive concepts that is easily confused or misunderstood. While it is about being in the *now* and *present moment*, mindfulness can seem invisible until you *know* it. And you can only really know it by *practicing* it, not by talking about it or thinking about it. Once you become mindful, your world changes. You become more aware and more focused on what is really happening around you. You begin to see and understand your fears and feelings around food much more clearly. To accomplish this, *Meal by Meal* uses daily themes that target your real world experience with food. With a theme for each day of the week –

Entry, Choices, Preparations, Rituals, Eating, Community, and Departure – you are guided gently and surely onto the path of mindfulness.

Eventually, you'll let go of the obstacles that keep you from enjoying the real purpose of food: to enhance the ultimate well-being of your mind, body, and spirit. What is more, when you gain the benefits of mindful eating, you also gain the benefits of mindful living. This translates into more peace around food and all stress in your life. It means understanding more deeply why and how you eat as you do. It means transforming your negative emotions and unskillful eating habits into more skillful ways of eating and being. My hope is that *Meal by Meal* helps you smile, savor, and explore food – without fear and worry – as the blessing it is meant to be in your life. In other words, may this book bring to you the beginning of a new way to taste and experience the bliss, balance, and healing potential of every bite.

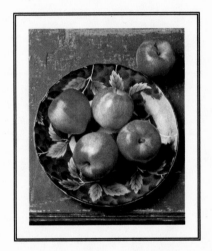

Entry

Lead me not into temptation;
I can find the way myself.

RITA MAE BROWN

EACH MEAL BRINGS EMOTIONAL CHALLENGES. Have you ever eaten a meal while you were angry, frustrated, or upset? Eat a meal in anger and you eat anger. Contemplate on this story before today's meal.

Two monks – one young and one elderly – gather food for their daily meal. On their way back to the monastery, a woman falls into the nearby river and struggles against the current. Without hesitation, the eldest monk carries her safely to the shore. The monks continue walking in silence until the young monk can no longer contain his anger.

"You carried that woman and broke your monk's vows."

"I left her on the bank," says the old monk. "But I am afraid you are still carrying her on your shoulders."

◆

Be mindful of your emotions
as you prepare to eat.

Choices

Fight your shame. Throw out your pride
and learn all you can from others. This is
the basis of a successful life.

SEN RIKYU, SIXTEENTH-CENTURY TEA MASTER

 YOUR MEALS REPRESENT A SERIES OF CHOICES.
Each choice is like a step that takes you in a particular direction. Over the years, similar choices, or habits, can lead you very far in one direction.

Ultimately, though, you are always free to choose another direction. You are always free to take a new step that is beyond habitual choice. Remember that healthy eating is also a habit and that change is always possible.

What one small achievable step can you take today? Even if you choose to eat one bite of a food that you think would be beneficial for you, it is enough for now. What would that food be? What foods not on your current "choice" list could contribute to your well-being?

◆

What new small choice would
you like to try today?

Preparations

Regard all utensils and goods of the
monastery as sacred vessels of the altar.
SAINT BENEDICT, *The Rule of St. Benedict*

 CLEANING THE KITCHEN CAN BE VIEWED AS AN onerous chore or approached as a way to cleanse and purify. Did you know that according to the Zen tradition, beginner monks are given easier chores while more experienced monks are given the most menial and demanding chores? Perhaps that is because the Zen masters know that it takes a special kind of wisdom (and person) to appreciate and learn from that which is most simple, plain, and uncluttered.

Watch your thoughts and attitudes as you clean your kitchen or any workspace. Can you let go of them for long enough to be in the moment with your task?

◆

Be mindful of even the simplest of tasks.

Rituals

No heaven can come to us unless our
hearts find rest in today. Take heaven!

FRA GIOVANNI, SIXTEENTH-CENTURY
ITALIAN ARCHITECT

WHEN YOU EAT FOR EMOTIONAL REASONS OR even out of boredom, it may be a sign that you seek greater meaning in your meals – and your life. Mealtime rituals offer fulfillment by showing you the divine nature and order of all things, visible and invisible.

This is illustrated in the story of a man who once searched for heaven on Earth.

"I have looked for angels," he said, "but I have yet to see one. I have looked for miracles, but never found anything worthy of God."

His neighbor, however, saw heaven everywhere he turned.

"I hear the angels singing in the wind that blows through the fields of wheat," he said, "and the miracle of God in each fruit and vegetable that sustains my life."

◆

Be mindful of the miracle of food
to sustain your life.

Eating

Patience ... moderation in food ...
[and] striving for spiritual advancements
is the teaching of all Buddhas.

THE BUDDHA

HAVE YOU EVER FOUND IT DIFFICULT TO EAT with patience and moderation? If so, you are not alone. And so you need to ask, what is patience with food? What does it mean to be moderate with food?

Buddha, for example, experienced both extremes of food. As a prince he ate to excess; as an ascetic he starved himself. Neither of them worked. Only after eating a moderate meal did he attain enlightenment. Thus, he learned the "middle way" that led to liberation.

The first step toward patience and moderation is simply watching and noticing when you are not patient and moderate. When you experience this, don't blame yourself. Instead, take a moment to consciously breathe in and out: Think "Creating a breath" as you slowly breathe in; think "Ending a breath" as you gently exhale. It's that simple to give yourself the gift of moderation and patience!

◆

Practice taking a breath in and a breath out
whenever you notice impatience.

Community

For it is in giving that we receive.

SAINT FRANCIS OF ASSISI, *A Simple Prayer*

 EACH MEAL, EACH MORSEL, IS A GIFT. EVEN IF you are single and eat many meals by yourself, that is why you never really eat alone. Consider for a moment, how each meal brings you into communion with the community at large.

The earth provides a bounty of food. Farmers plant seeds and harvest crops. Truckers transport food to local distribution centers. Retailers stock the shelves.

This great chain of being and giving never ends. That you are part of a community and a planet that share food is one of the amazing gifts of being. In the broader sense, is not each meal – indeed, everything in your life – something that is given? This is true even when you work for your meals – because even one's livelihood can be viewed as a blessing.

◆

Be mindful that each foodstuff connects us
to our planet and our community.

Departure

May peace be with you.

AS ONE MEAL ENDS, ANOTHER JOURNEY BEGINS. What kind of energy fills your body after your meal? Are you drowsy? Alert? Anxious? Guilty? Pay attention to how different food affects your body. Over time you can become more skillful at making choices that help you transition to your "after-meal" stage more easily.

Remember, too, that you eat thousands of meals in a lifetime. There is no one perfect meal for you. However, there are many more meals at which you can make adjustments. Accept your meal and the choices you make today. It is enough to be aware of what you feel at this moment.

As you become aware of your thoughts and opinions on your meal, take a conscious breath. Now, rest with compassion for today's choices, and bring compassion to your next meal.

◆

Be at peace with the meal
you have just eaten.

Entry

Waiting is a state of mind. Basically, it means that
you want the future; you don't want the present.

ECKHART TOLLE, *The Power of Now*

THE SUBTLE FEELINGS YOU HAVE ABOUT YOUR next meal can cause you to feel anxiety, anticipation, excitement, fear, calm, and even peace. As you await your next meal, what is your state of mind? If you are not sure, pause for a moment as you make your way to the next meal. Take a breath and feel any restriction in your breath, body, or mind.

Sometimes feelings are subtle, like gently shifting wind. Let yourself sense the breeze within. You can rest in the knowledge that you don't need to push away any feelings about food or eating. When you push something away, does it often push back even harder? If you are fearful of eating, for example, let yourself sense your fear.

With self-knowledge of your eating emotions, you gain a measure of peace and self-mastery. Simply acknowledge that this is what you feel at this moment. To do this is to live with grace and self-acceptance at a deep level.

◆

Acknowledge and accept your emotions
without judgment or pushing them away.

Choices

*As a child my family's menu consisted
of two choices: take it or leave it.*

BUDDY HACKETT

MANY TIMES, MEMORIES OF CHILDHOOD FOODS can stay with you – and even subconsciously affect your food choices. Do you remember the foods you ate when you were growing up? The ones you liked and the ones you hated? These memories may cause you to gravitate toward certain foods and avoid others. That is why it is helpful to think about how food choices change over time.

For example, take a moment to think about the foods you ate as a child, a teenager, a young adult, and finally, as an adult. Whether or not you are journaling, it may be helpful to notice the change in food choices over these four stages. What foods are different? What foods remain the same? Look at the overall pattern. Simply observe the clues as a detective might – no blame, no shame.

◆

Create a "food inventory" and
acknowledge that you have the freedom
to change your eating habits.

Preparations

Intention combined with detachment leads to
life-centered, present-moment awareness.

DEEPAK CHOPRA, *The Seven Spiritual Laws of Success*

ANYTIME YOU PREPARE TO COOK – EVEN IF IT is to put a TV dinner in the oven or microwave – you first set an intention. When you think about it, do you not set an intention before almost anything? Can you imagine, for example, sitting down to eat if you had no intention to do so? The act of eating would be empty. But if you are hungry, and you set the intention to eat a nourishing and satisfying meal, then you will be fully engaged and savor it. The same is true of preparation.

Intention during preparation is an important step in mealtime mindfulness. It means you are putting your attention on what you are about to do – right now in the present moment. You are not thinking about the appointment you just had or about tomorrow's shopping list. Keep reminding yourself of your intention to prepare a meal – whether the meal is for yourself or for others.

◆

Set an intention to prepare your meal, and
experience how it changes the preparation.

Rituals

The fruit of silence is prayer,
The fruit of prayer is faith,
The fruit of faith is love and
The fruit of love is silence.

MOTHER TERESA

A RITUAL PRAYER – BEFORE, DURING, OR AFTER a meal – can transform eating and food from the mundane to the sacred. Sometimes it is useful to think about your own history of ritual. As a child, did your family have a mealtime ritual? How was it structured? Most importantly, how did you feel about it? Did the process feel forced? Or was it filled with love and acceptance? Or, if you had no ritual, how do you feel about that now?

However you may have experienced it, how you decide to use ritual in the present is up to you. You have the freedom to shape and transform a mealtime ritual that fits your needs and sensibilities. Whether you live by yourself, as a single parent, with a partner, or as part of a larger family unit, meaningful ritual can add richness and togetherness to ordinary meals. It acknowledges the mystery of food, the awesome wonder of how it nourishes and allows you to reach your life dreams and goals.

◆

Reflect on the specific feeling
and meaning you would like in a ritual
designed especially for you.

Eating

Tea is nought but this:
First you heat the water,
Then you make the tea.
Then you drink it properly,
That is all you need to know.

SEN RIKYU, SIXTEENTH-CENTURY TEA MASTER

 DID YOU EVER EXPERIENCE A TEA CEREMONY? I once had the opportunity to attend a full-fledged Japanese tea ceremony that consisted of thick tea, or *matcha*, thin tea, and a complete meal. Traditionally, the tea ceremony is very ceremonial, with special ways of handling utensils and wiping off the tea cup, and so on. Honestly, I was worried that I would embarrass myself and the host. However, my fears were unfounded.

Tea, like any meal, only asks that you be aware of each little movement of your body and everything before you. This is mindfulness, and with this little secret you can find moment-to-moment oneness with anything – especially food. While you eat, simply pay attention. Mindfulness uses bare awareness to just watch. With bare awareness, a banana is not yellow, curved, and sweet. It just is. Use bare awareness and mindfulness to experience food in a fresh, new way.

◆

With bare awareness, observe your eating.

Community

A kitchen condenses the universe.

BETTY FUSSELL, *My Kitchen Wars*

THE JOURNEY OF FOOD BEGINS LONG BEFORE IT appears sanitized, frozen, processed, prepared, and packaged neatly on your grocery shelves. Food all begins alive, in the world, swimming in rivers and oceans, grazing on ranches, growing on trees, and ripening in fields. Too often we think of food just as any manufactured product, when in truth it is of the earth, like all of us. If you really think about it, the wholeness of food is dependent on an entire community that is responsible for getting food on our table.

Then, there are those who distribute and ship the food to our local communities. The effort is massive and seamless, which is why it is easy for us – unlike countries less fortunate – to take our bounty for granted.

◆

Reflect on the individuals who
made your meal possible, and appreciate
them and the earth that sustains life.

Departure

*When the pain of loneliness comes
upon you, confront it, look at it without
any thought of running away.*

KRISHNAMURTI, *Think on These Things*

FOR SOME, LEAVING A MEAL CAN MEAN DEPARTING from what is secure, comforting, and familiar. Have you ever left a meal with a sense of emptiness and emotional hunger?

I can recall a time in my own life, shortly after graduating from college, when I ate comfort food (rice pudding) every day one summer to ease the pain of loneliness. Unfortunately, as soon as I finished eating, I was alone again with my thoughts and my pain.

You may adopt a strict diet plan as a way to ignore uncomfortable feelings about your emotions or body. But pushing your feelings underground only allows them to hide in waiting, ready to ambush you by causing you to lose control of that diet. Better to give feelings a voice and make friends with them. In the long run, this is how to heal food cravings.

◆

Be mindful of your feelings
after you finish your meal.

Entry

*Every new cycle of growth, every
step we take toward a deeper realization of self,
every death and rebirth of our current and future
identity adds a wonderful sheen to our veneer,
to our character . . . to our crust.*

BROTHER PETER REINHART,
Brother Juniper's Bread Book

WHAT IS THE "CRUST" OF EMOTIONAL ENERGY you bring with you to today's meal? Are you excited to gain sustenance and meaning? Or are you tired and worn out, just going through the motions of eating?

It helps to understand where you are in your own personal cycle of growth. You, like all of nature, possess a season, a time for growth and expending energy or a time for slowing down and repose. There is a time for holding on, and a time for letting go.

If you have been pushing your body and mind hard at work, for example, consider how that will affect your food choices and experience. Does your body need more food or less? What kind of food does your body truly desire at this moment? Take a conscious breath and slow down. Listen deeply.

◆

Breathe mindfully and become aware
of your personal season and emotions as you
enter the space for your next meal.

Choices

The path is easy for those who have no preferences.

Sanaya Roman, *Spiritual Growth*

 Have your food choices ever caused you pain and suffering? This could have something to do with how strongly attached you are to your choices. There is a big difference, for example, between obsessions and preferences.

Obsessions are very strong, singular desires, ideas, or beliefs that have become inflexible and rigid – even if they can cause you harm. I know of a woman who had only chocolate bars in her refrigerator. She offered many reasons why this made sense, but actually, she wanted a better way to feed her hunger with a healthy balance of nutrients.

Does that mean that passionately loving chocolate is bad? Preferences represent a choice that permits adaptation and change. So if chocolate is not available, then maybe a piece of fruit will do. By contrast, a singular, or obsessive, point of view – about vegetables, chocolate, or any idea – blocks out your choices and limits your freedom.

◆

Pay attention to your food preferences
today. How flexible or inflexible are they?

Preparations

*To be blind is bad, but worse
it is to have eyes and not to see.*

HELEN KELLER

CLOSE YOUR EYES FOR A MOMENT. CAN YOU VISU-
alize your cooking and preparation space? Whether your
kitchen is large or small, try to identify where everything is without looking. Now think about that space in more detail. Is everything you need to prepare a meal easy to find? Are spices and
ingredients where you can find them? Or do you have to dig through
cabinets looking for each one? Then there is your preparation space.
Is it cluttered or open? Inviting or limiting?

Preparation begins with mindfulness of your working space –
whether you are a chef building a salad in your kitchen or simply
heating leftovers in the microwave. It is easier and more fun to prepare when your space is clean and uncluttered. The result is perhaps
fewer spills and accidents, and a tastier meal.

♦

Think about how you would rearrange
your kitchen space to make preparation
easier and more fun. (Optional: Do it!)

Rituals

Do not turn away what is given you,
nor reach out for what is given to others,
lest you disturb your quietness.

THE BUDDHA, *Dhammapada*

ALL THAT WE HAVE IN OUR KITCHEN – FROM the food in the refrigerator to the dishes and condiments in the cabinets – has been offered from some worldly source. Have you ever heard of the traditional Native American ritual called the "giveaway"? This is a vital ritual through which individuals can experience the extent of giving that exists in their lives and their world. The giveaway asks, first and foremost, that we acknowledge that what we have has all been given to us.

Think about this. Even though we pay for the meal we eat in a restaurant, it still was created for our benefit. The giveaway asks that we gain the maturity to recognize and be grateful for this, then to give something back. Is this the season of your life to return something?

◆

During your meal, recall memorable
food giveaways – currently or in the past –
that have blessed your life.

Eating

*Giving up smoking is the easiest thing
in the world. I know because I've done it
thousands of times.*

MARK TWAIN

IS THERE A FOOD HABIT YOU REALLY, REALLY want to change? The power of desire can keep us frozen in habitual behavior. So, what is the secret to changing any habit? The first step is acknowledging and accepting our own habits without trying to judge them. This acceptance and tolerance for our inner desires is a starting point from which to make a change.

Remember that food change cannot be forced. We must invite it into our lives as a friend. We must get to know it intimately. Only then can we take the next steps – forgiveness and a vow to change. But it is always worthwhile to revisit acceptance. One beneficial and powerful method is to recognize "food static" in our lives. This can be tempting food at the market, advertisements, and even those cookies (metaphorical or literal) that confront us during the holidays or at other times.

◆

Become aware of food static
all around you as you pay attention to
your inner reactions and desires.

Community

*To truly listen to another is a main course
of the family's inner meal.*

DONALD ALTMAN, *Art of the Inner Meal*

MEALS CAN HEAL. WHEN YOU WERE A CHILD, did you have a chance to speak freely, to contribute, to have a voice and be heard at mealtime? Even if you were not so fortunate, such is the potential of a healing meal. To truly listen to those who matter most is to witness and understand your family's – or your community's – story.

If you eat with others, then you can gain the skill to heal by letting them be heard. But where do you begin? The first step, as with all mindfulness, is to gain awareness of what is. Just observe and learn. Is everyone fighting for the last word? Is everyone debating with the need to be right? Or maybe no one speaks except to say, "pass the potatoes."

If you eat alone, you can also open yourself to the sounds of what is around you at mealtime. Listening is both a gift and a birthright. Be spacious, kind, and forgiving of whatever you witness.

✦

Take a calming, mindful breath-in
and breath-out as you let others speak
without interrupting, and observe
interactions at mealtime.

Departure

It's not what you're eating. It's what's eating you.

ANONYMOUS

IS SOMETHING UPSETTING YOU WHILE YOU EAT? If so, you are not alone. What and how you eat can affect your mood. After all, it is not just what you eat that matters. *How* you eat affects your feelings. A meal eaten in haste and anxiety can naturally cause you to carry those feelings with you after you leave the table. If you are dissatisfied or unhappy after your meal, for example, do you ever take that feeling with you – to your next meeting or environment?

Sometimes, the feelings you experience after eating are physical. Overeating, for example, may make you sluggish and tired. Eating a particular type of food – such as turkey – may cause drowsiness. In a food journal, note how you feel after mealtime. Look for differences between times when you feel a sense of well-being and times when you do not.

♦

Pay attention to how you feel –
emotionally and physically – after your meal.

Entry

Your karma is in the refrigerator.

DONALD ALTMAN, *Art of the Inner Meal*

Do you often go to the refrigerator or the convenience store without really knowing what you want to eat? You can practice "refrigerator mindfulness" by taking stock of your reactions. Allow yourself to experience three types of mindfulness: (1) your sensations, (2) your mind/perceptions, and (3) your body.

Sensations include your awareness of taste, sight, touch, smell, and sound, as well as whether the feeling you get is pleasant, unpleasant, or neutral. Food is powerful because eating engages all of your feelings through the five senses! The second type of mindfulness is mind/perceptions, which includes your bare awareness, plus the personal perceptions you add to it – desires, cravings, opinions, and emotions. Lastly, mindfulness encompasses the physical form, such as posture and your body's reaction to the food – or to anything.

Begin refrigerator mindfulness by limiting yourself to one type of mindfulness at a time: your sensations, mind/perceptions, or body. You need not react, but just experience whatever is present in your body, mind, and thoughts.

✦

Practice refrigerator mindfulness by opening
the door and experiencing the three distinct
types of mindfulness.

Choices

For months the fool may fast, eating from the tip
of a grass blade. Still he is not worth a penny beside
the master, whose food is the way.

THE BUDDHA, *Dhammapada*

HAVE YOU EVER STRUGGLED WITH CONTROLLING your food choices or the quantity of food you eat? If so, then you are in good company. That is because the Buddha, Jesus, and others learned that food moderation was vital to health and spiritual growth. Jesus revolted against the strict food laws of his time by saying, "There is nothing outside a man which by going into him can defile him; but the things which come out of a man are what defile him." The Buddha gave up fasting for the "middle way" of eating in moderation – and shortly after attained enlightenment.

You may be doing yourself a disservice by defining yourself so narrowly by what you eat – thereby creating separations between yourself and others, when compassion would be the wiser course.

◆

Witness your limiting, constricted
ideas about food choices. As you do so,
forgive yourself for choices that may have
been harmful or extreme.

Preparations

Crack the egg of ignorance.

Nyishöl Khenpo Rinpoche, Tibetan Buddhist

THE ENTIRE PROCESS OF COOKING AND PREPA-
RAtion is all about change. Bread turns into toast. An un-
adorned head of lettuce, a hard-boiled egg, and a tomato become
a fresh salad. Butter, wine, and spices transform into an elegant
sauce.

How we go about this makes all the difference. For that reason,
I say this: We are all eggs waiting to be cracked. That is because
each time we prepare food, our thin outer shells are opened to the
space of uncertainty.

We know that the results and outcome of placing a frozen dinner in the microwave cannot always be predicted! Nor should they
be. Let the space of preparation open us to unexpected creativity and
growth. Accept this uncertainty with compassion.

◆

Open yourself to uncertainty and release
expectations during preparation.

Rituals

In joy or sadness, flowers are our constant friends.
We eat, drink, sing, dance, and flirt with them.
We wed and christen with them.

KAKUZO OKAKURA, *The Book of Tea*

IS THERE SOMETHING SPECIAL THAT ACCOMPANIES your mealtime? Sometimes the rituals in your life are so ingrained and invisible that you may not even recognize them. Whether you eat by yourself or with others, "invisible" rituals that enrich your mealtime include such things as music, a vase of flowers, even a lit candle.

There are also unspoken mealtime rituals that touch you every day. In many Asian countries, for example, the eldest is served the food before anyone else gets a chance to fill his or her plate. Even the Western practice of waiting for others to be seated and served before eating is a ritual that declares a sense of order and meaning.

Rituals offer you a comforting familiarity that helps to feel normal, even when you may be coping with stress or experiencing difficulties. By adding personal ritual to your meal, you imbue it with a richness that fulfills at many levels.

◆

Add a new ritual – flowers, music,
and grace – to one of your meals.

Eating

I call on a dream that reminds us to focus on our
fingertips, on the shape and weight of our hand,
on blood and bone and a thousand nerve endings
as we raise an apple to our mouths.

ORIAH MOUNTAIN DREAMER, AUTHOR

HAVE YOU EVER FORGOTTEN A MEAL SHORTLY after you ate it? Fortunately, mindfulness focuses the attention on every little detail of sight, taste, movement, smell, and sound. This way, you can never forget how miraculous it is to simply bite into an apple!

An entire network of interconnected synapses navigates your hand with its sensitive nerves toward the apple. Your optic nerve sends upside-down images of the apple to the brain (where the images are translated). Your olfactory senses are some of the body's most ancient sensing equipment. And your taste buds send messages to your pleasure centers as the hearing apparatus picks up the vibrations of your chewing.

Then, of course, there are the myriad involuntary systems that work simultaneously, enabling you to breathe and digest as you eat your meal. Revel in this master orchestration the next time you bite an apple.

◆

Be aware of all your body's
actions in a single bite.

Community

*Storytelling is a way of giving someone
great and lasting wealth.*

JOSEPH BRUCHAC, NATIVE AMERICAN
STORYTELLER AND AUTHOR

CHANCES ARE, YOU HAVE HEARD (AND SHARED) some fascinating stories with others over food. Isn't this a good way to get to know another? In truth, we are constantly telling and retelling the story of who we are – as a global community, a country, a culture, a city, a neighborhood, a family, and as individuals.

For example, history (his-story) contains many perspectives and myths. Is any single version correct? Don't you get a more complete story when you share and hear all sides of another's situation? Even if you eat dinner alone while watching TV, you can watch the news or any show from a more spacious point of view.

While your experience of life is unique, you share the universal experience of living on this planet with others – of sharing Earth's gifts of air and food in order to survive. At mealtime, listen to the story of others with a great and open heart. In doing so, you learn more about the story of us all.

◆

Share your story, and let others
share theirs without judgment.

Departure

True acceptance is saying,
"It's all right, it's all right, it's all right."

EMMANUEL, *Emmanuel's Book*

HAVE YOU EVER EATEN AT AN "ALL YOU CAN EAT" buffet? Chances are that either you or someone you know has been tempted to eat more than normal. When this happens, how accepting are you of your actions? Have you ever said to yourself, "That proves I can't control my eating," or "I have zero willpower and can't stay on a diet"? At times like this you need to remember that this is only one meal and no crime has been committed!

Acceptance is like a salve that heals your self-inflicted wounds. It gives you kindness and compassion when you can find none. Is there anyone who has not struggled with eating at one time or another? All physical beings struggle for and with food. Only you can forgive the unforgiving voice within.

◆

Rest with compassion and
acceptance, and forgive yourself for
meals eaten mindlessly.

Entry

You have reproved me for eating very little, but
I only eat to live, whereas you live to eat.

SOCRATES

How do you think your diet affects your overall health and longevity? In the twenty-first century, we pride ourselves on our ever-increasing life expectancy. But many of us may be surprised to learn that the Buddha lived until age eighty, when he died of food poisoning from tainted boar's flesh. Socrates also lived until eighty, when his life ended prematurely because he was forced to drink hemlock. Aristotle and Plato lived to ninety years of age!

How did people who lived more than 2000 years ago – with no antibiotics – maintain active lives for so long? Given modern medicine, our present-day life expectancy should be 150 years or more.

Many ancient Greeks subsisted on a modest diet of unfired vegetables. This confirms what many traditions tell us: seasonal and local foods may be the most harmonious for our bodies. And, Socrates' practice of moderation in eating seems to have contributed to his long life.

❖

Pay attention to how much you eat,
and how much food you really need.

Choices

The food is brahma (creative energy).
Its essence is vishnu (preservative energy).
The eater is shiva (destructive energy).
No sickness due to food can come
To one who eats with this knowledge.

SANSKRIT BLESSING

 WHENEVER WE EAT, WE ABSORB THE ENERGY essence of food. Has food ever made you drowsy, excitable, or calm? According to ancient Hindu beliefs, for example, all physical matter is formed by the condensed vibratory energy of the cosmos. This energy takes three basic forms, which we absorb when we eat. The first energy is called *tamas*, which has qualities that cause us to become tired, lazy, slow, weak, and dull. The next, *rajas*, possesses qualities that cause increased heat, ambition, hunger, and emotion. The remaining energy, *sattva*, fills us with balance, harmony, composure, and spiritual lightness.

Now, reflect on foods that cause us to lose energy and hinder our progress. Think about those that stimulate. Also, ponder those that generate a feeling of well-being and harmony. As the adage says, "You are what you eat."

◆

Tune in to the amazing changes that
come from absorbing the energy of each
different food. Journal these feelings.

Preparations

*If you simply read the recipes without
putting them into practice, it's like knowing
about peppers, onions, and garlic, but never
knowing how they taste.*

RONNA KABATZNICK, *The Zen of Eating*

DO YOU EVER FEEL NERVOUS OR SCATTERED WHEN planning or making a meal? Mindfulness can soothe mealtime emotions. For this daily meditation, you will spend some practice time walking around your kitchen or other living space. When I spent time in a monastery, for example, I would always take a twenty-minute walking meditation outside before breakfast.

Begin by simply resting in place, breathing slowly. Now make the intention "to take a step with my right foot," and as you do so, follow up with that action. Observe the movement of your leg as it steps. Next, make the intention "to take a step with my left foot," and take that step. Over and over, make intentions followed by action and observation. Feel everything – your judgments (this is too slow, boring, fascinating, etc.), your body, your awareness. Step as quickly or slowly as your intention lets you for 1 to 3 minutes, or until you feel centered and balanced. Carry that feeling with you into preparation.

◆

Experience a mindful walk around your
living space before food preparation.

Rituals

The spiritual journey does not
require going anywhere because God is
already with us and in us.

FATHER THOMAS KEATING, *Open Mind, Open Heart*

FOLLOWING THE ADVICE OF FATHER THOMAS KEATING, ritual merely opens the door to what is already present at mealtime – or anytime. If you want to feel the depth of your experience, you need to be honest and open. For, as Shakespeare once wrote, "To thine own self be true."

The key here is to open up to the potential of your connection to spirit and others. Before saying your ritual blessing, give yourself permission to feel the divine presence around you – in whatever form it may take.

If you feel frustrated or bored, let that be your experience of the divine at mealtime. If you feel moved or elated, then that can be your experience. Allow yourself the space to feel differently at each meal. Your mealtime ritual journey is a process, not an end point.

◆

Reflect on your truth toward
food and others during a meal.

Eating

We learn speech from men, silence from the gods.

PLUTARCH

HAVE YOU EVER CONSCIOUSLY EATEN A MEAL in silence? This practice has been a part of many monastic practices for centuries. One reason why this is useful is that you can more easily focus attention on your meal and on the mindfulness surrounding it, such as your breath.

Do you breathe while you eat? When I ask this question of participants in my Mindful and Sacred Eating Workshops, many of them have no idea. Silence makes it easier to concentrate on how you breathe, chew, and swallow and how the taste and texture of food changes in your mouth. It even lets you focus on how certain flavors fill you with desire for more food.

Try this with your silence: Take a breath between each bite. Chew twenty times or more before swallowing.

◆

Experience silence, breathing,
and chewing during meals.

Community

First, do no harm.

HIPPOCRATES

THE GREEK DOCTOR HIPPOCRATES, WHO IS CON-
sidered the father of medicine, developed the first medical
code of ethics, known as the Hippocratic oath. His admonition
Do no harm is central in all traditions and is vital to how we relate
to our community. So then, how can we do no harm at mealtime?

First, we can take steps to ensure that our meal does not become a battlefield where anger and negative emotion boil over. This
does not mean we should cover up our feelings. What it does mean,
though, is that we can try to show respect and patience toward
those we share a meal with. This is not always easy. Patience and forbearance are in danger of becoming lost arts. To practice them is to
sow the seeds of peace and non-harm at mealtime. Even if we eat
alone, we need patience and forbearance for ourselves – this is also
a form of non-harm that lessens our own mental battles.

◆

Bring patience and forbearance
into your meal.

Departure

There is a time for departure,
even when there's no certain place to go.

TENNESSEE WILLIAMS

DO YOU EVER FIND IT DIFFICULT TO BID FAREWELL after an enjoyable meal? If so, you might appreciate the farewell celebration for the Chinese kitchen god that takes place on February 4. Traditionally, many Chinese leave offerings of salty fish or sticky sweet cakes for the kitchen god who returns to heaven to report on each family's behavior. A good report results in bountiful cupboards in the year to come.

If you were a kitchen god, what report would you make about your mealtime farewell behavior? Do you hold on to mealtime sights, sounds, and tastes? Do you constantly replay dinner conversation or wish that you had done things differently?

It is normal to remember mealtime events. But a mindful departure means being present here and now. This lets you exit gracefully, not overstay your welcome. Staying is easy. Leaving is an art.

◆

Observe how you hold on after
departing your meal. Each time you find
yourself holding on, gently let go.

Entry

When the flower blooms, the bees come uninvited.

RAMAKRISHNA,
NINETEENTH-CENTURY HINDU SAGE

IF YOU DO NOT FEEL YOUR HUNGER BUT FIND you eat anyway, it may help to follow nature's example. A flower blooms when it must. A rain cloud rains without wondering whether it will ruin someone's picnic. Each flower, each blade of grass, moves to the ticking and beat of its own time clock.

Humans also have natural rhythms. Let your rhythms guide you and help you more naturally discover when you are hungry – not emotionally hungry, but physically hungry.

The number of meals eaten daily varies from culture to culture. Our society tells us three meals a day at set times are the norm. But what is best for you? When does your hunger blossom?

Generally, though, do not skip breakfast. A healthy early meal signals your body that you are active. In fact, eating less can make weight loss more difficult because the body slows your metabolism to conserve energy.

◆

Let yourself feel when you are
really hungry. Can you adjust some
of your meals to those times?

Choices

Whenever I make a choice, I will ask myself two
questions: "What are the consequences of this
choice that I am making?" and "Will this choice
bring fulfillment and happiness to me and also to
those who are affected by this choice?"

DEEPAK CHOPRA, *The Seven Spiritual Laws of Success*

 WHEN YOU HEAR THE WORD "ECOSYSTEM," WHAT
do you think about? Actually, there are many different
ecosystems. Your body, for instance, is a self-contained, incredibly
efficient ecosystem. Your lungs are like the air, your blood like the
rivers and streams. What food is best to maintain your personal
ecosystem in balance and harmony?

Bear in mind that the choices you make for your personal ecosystem also have an impact on the world's ecosystem. What is the
impact on the planet of raising cattle or growing genetically modified cereals and grains? There are many books written on these
topics, such as Francis Moore Lappé's *Diet for a Small Planet*. I am
not saying that you should stop eating beef. However, it benefits
you to become more aware of your food choices – for yourself,
your children, and all beings.

◆

What impact do your food choices have
on the planet and your well-being?

Preparations

*The trouble with ordinary reality is that
a lot of it is dull, so we long ago decided to
leave for somewhere better.*

CHARLES TART, *Living the Mindful Life*

DO YOU OFTEN CHECK OUT DURING KITCHEN preparation and cleaning? Is your mind miles away on a fantasy trip?

Really, it is not that ordinary reality is so dull – we just do not pay enough attention to it to see how impressive and fresh it can really be! There is an ancient Zen phrase, "Chop wood; carry water," that leads us to where the action is. It is right here, in front of us.

While chopping a lettuce, for example, we can engage the power of attention to bring us into the moment. We can feel the weight of the knife and the crispness of the produce – all while mindfully following through with the action and observing the results. Each time we get to a new step, we can use intention, observation, and action to enter each fresh moment.

✦

Stay mindful during meal preparation.

Rituals

However many holy words you read,
however many you speak, what good will they do
if you do not act upon them?

THE BUDDHA

WITH THIS ADVICE, THE BUDDHA COULD HAVE been invoking the popular slogan Just do it. You invite the sacred into your home and your meal by doing more than just reciting the words of grace. The real objective is to make those words real, to transform them into action, and to manifest them in the world.

Suppose that your mealtime grace includes the idea of thankfulness for the food on your plate. You can naturally extend that thankfulness out into the world by inviting that lonely neighbor to your house for dinner. Maybe you could take part in offering food to others. There are many programs for donating or delivering food, such as Meals-on-Wheels, that help you share your thankfulness and your bounty. Just one thing, even a little thing, is a great place to start!

◆

What can I do to bring my blessings
into the world?

Eating

Life can only be created by life; health only
comes from an integration of our various levels
of function – not from the intake of
manufactured pills and potions.

ANNEMARIE COLBIN, *Food and Healing*

OUR BODIES ARE NOT MACHINES, ALTHOUGH WE sometimes think of them in a mechanistic way. Rather, I like to think of the body as a divine vehicle holding the inseparable parts of our physical form (body), mind, and spirit. Tugging on the strings of any one cannot help but move the others. If we ingest food that is not beneficial for our body, then it will likewise affect the ability of our mind and spirit to operate optimally.

Spiritual teachers know that food – as well as breath, exercises, prayer, and fasting – can be used to attain spiritual growth. That is why it helps to make a list of those foods we think would be our "ideal diet" for mind, body, and spirit.

◆

Add a new "ideal" food to your diet today.

Community

The brothers should serve one another.
Consequently, no one will be excused from kitchen
service unless he is sick or engaged in some
important business of the monastery, for such
service increases reward and fosters love.

SAINT BENEDICT, *The Rule of St. Benedict*

 PERSONALLY, I TRY TO MAKE A POINT OF HELPING to clean up at mealtime. Even when I am a guest, I offer my assistance. That was not always the case, however. When I was in high school, I considered cleaning up a chore worthy only of avoidance. Only now do I recognize the wisdom of parents who have their children take on responsibility around the kitchen or home.

For example, the idea of taking responsibility is an integral part of the tea ceremony. The whole idea behind tea is to create mindfulness between host and guest. Therefore, the idea of respect is highly valued and practiced.

When we respect others we value them and take our share of the load. Adapt respect and responsibility as part of your family values and experience the change it makes.

◆

Reflect on your responsibilities as a
way of showing respect and love for your
family and community.

Departure

If we live in mindfulness, we are no longer
poor, because our practice of living in the
present moment makes us rich in joy, peace,
understanding, and love.

THICH NHAT HANH, *Our Appointment with Life*

ONE POSITIVE WAY TO EXPERIENCE MINDFULNESS after mealtime is to take a walk. The Buddha recommended this over 2500 years ago. The Greek doctor Hippocrates also recommended exercise for long life. Of course, this is contrary to the words of the comedian who once commented, "Every time I feel the urge to exercise, I lie down." The choice is yours, but once you try mindful walking you may decide to make it more of a healthy habit after eating.

While mindful walking is often done slowly, you can also walk quickly or briskly if that fits your style. If you do the brisk walk, just breathe normally and focus on your body and movements as you walk. Stay present, always aware of your balance and your breath.

◆

Be mindful after your meal with a short walk.

Entry

*You might be the most depressed person in the
world, the most addicted person in the world,
the most jealous person in the world . . . All of that
is a good place to start.*

Pema Chödrön, *Start Where You Are*

WHAT IS YOUR MOST DIFFICULT EATING ISSUE?
Do you eat too much? Do you eat less than is good for you?
Are you rigid with your choices? Are you addicted to potato chips,
ice cream, or some other food? Do you beat yourself up emotionally for eating the things you think you "shouldn't"? Think of your
worst food problem, and you have just found the best place for you
to start.

Thinking about where you "should" be often creates an obstacle. This "should" thought gets you (and many of us) into trouble,
because it focuses on your guilt and blame rather than on accepting the joyful truth of your starting place. Only by starting where
you are and by being mindful of your emotional hunger can you
truly deal with any issue or the pain surrounding it.

◆

Where is your best, most honest place from
which to start healing?

Choices

*What other people think about me is none
of my business.*

JOHN BENASSU, PSYCHOTHERAPIST

HOW MUCH AND WHAT YOU PUT INTO YOUR
mouth is your own business. You cannot blame others for
your choices. Neither can you worry what others will think of your
choices. What you can do, however, is take responsibility for what
is on your plate, then accept and forgive yourself.

When you think about it, you are supposed to be choosing exactly the foods that are on your plate right now! All the choices
you have made up over the years have created a habitual style of
eating – a pattern of likes and dislikes. All of this predicts what
you will likely eat at your next meal. Do not expect that you can
easily change this pattern in a day, a week, or a month.

Only by ever so slowly making a new choice here, a new choice
there, can you establish a new pattern and the freedom to choose.
Change your food and health karma one choice at a time. Make
even one skillful choice today, and leave the blame game to someone else.

◆

Reflect on how others impact your choices,
then choose one food that is beneficial
for you, regardless of others.

Preparations

Give me the provisions and whole apparatus
of a kitchen, and I would starve.

MONTAIGNE

NOT EVERYONE IS AT HOME WITH A BLENDER
or food processor. Whatever your feelings or awkwardness
about preparation, you can begin simply by working with basic
cooking instruments and utensils. Some years ago I attended a professional chef's class. I was very much a novice in a class filled with
people who ran restaurants and owned catering businesses. That did
not stop me from learning.

I remember learning how to roll my French-crafted chef's knife
in a graceful up and down motion that quickly diced any vegetable
to size. To this day, there is something musical and poetic about
the rhythmic sound of the blade tapping on a wooden cutting board.
I have kept and cared for that wonderful cutlery.

There is no shame in learning about food, and sometimes the
fundamentals are the most fun.

♦

Learn a new preparation technique or
discover how to use a new utensil.

Rituals

Your spirit is mixing with my spirit just as wine
is mixing with pure water. And when something
touches you, it touches me. Now "you" are
"me" in everything!

AL-HALLAJ, TENTH-CENTURY
MYSTIC AND SUFI MASTER

 RITUALS CAN SOMETIMES BE SOLEMN AND SERI-
ous. But they can just as easily be brimming with a sense
of joy, lightness, and laughter. Did you know, for example, that during the Jewish Sabbath, it is considered sinful to worry or be sad?
That is why the Sabbath is typically accompanied with song and
music. The table setting is beautified with good linen, plates, and
utensils. And the participants dress up in their best clothes.

This makes sense when you realize that the ritual Sabbath represents a shift from the ordinary working week and mundane living into a spiritual dimension. Here, all that matters is the present
moment of communion with family and the divine. I know of one
family, for example, that created its own ritual meal – complete
with candles, singing, a blessing, and beautified table setting. You
can do the same.

✦

Think about inviting your family
or community to share in creating a
special ritual meal.

Eating

Mindfulness is free. We are born with it.

VENERABLE U SILANANDA,
BURMESE MONK AND TEACHER

I STILL REMEMBER THE MORNING I WAS TOLD TO sit opposite the head of the monastery during lunch. This was an honor, but I was mildly alarmed. What worried me was that U Silananda had written a well-known book about mindfulness. I was positive he would see my unsteady mind and mindless eating habits. But once I sat at the table, I decided to slow down and simply eat as if I already knew how to be mindful rather than be concerned about him being across the table. It worked.

One of the things I appreciate most about mindfulness is that it is not only about our own eating. Mindfulness extends to those we are with. The monks I shared meals with always watched to see when someone needed more rice or food. We, too, can be grateful and attentive to everything happening around us – even if we happen to be dining alone.

◆

Eat a meal as if you were already
a mindfulness master.

Community

We need myths that will identify the individual
not with his local group but with the planet.
JOSEPH CAMPBELL, *The Power of Myth*

EATING IS NOT JUST ABOUT GULPING DOWN today's meal. There is a bigger picture to be found in the mythic journey of food. Myth is present in all life, and food is another mythic journey that we all travel. Discovering your universal journey regarding food may offer new insight into your life.

As a mythic food traveler, you answer a call – which might be anything from struggling with a diet to overcoming an illness. The movie *Star Wars*, for example, tapped into the power of the mythic journey. When you decide to face and answer your call – as Luke Skywalker did – you, too, become a hero.

While you alone take your hero's journey, you can broaden your view and gain strength by expanding the people you share your meals with. Just think of the famous cantina scene in *Star Wars*, where aliens of every shape and kind are drinking and eating.

◆

Reflect on your journey with food and eating.
What is the "call" that you are undertaking?

Departure

I do not think that anything serious should be done
after dinner, as nothing should be before breakfast.

GEORGE SAINTSBURY,
TWENTIETH-CENTURY BRITISH CRITIC

HOW CAN YOU MAKE A GRACEFUL TRANSITION from mealtime? How can you settle yourself down, without the pressure to immediately jump back on life's treadmill?

In many countries it is common to take a siesta after lunch. Why is this? It is probably because the body is busy digesting the meal. That is one reason, for example, that I advise against meditating after eating. Similarly, swimming after a meal is also not recommended. Some writers do not like to work on a full stomach since the blood rushes from the head to the stomach to digest the meal. And so, you need to recognize how digestion alters your body and mind.

If a siesta is not accepted at your workplace, find a few moments of solitude where you can close your eyes. Or take a short, calming nature walk. You might try to transition with a cup of tea or some soothing music before becoming active again.

◆

Seek peace after mealtime; make a gentle
transition to activity.

Entry

Man shall not live by bread alone, but by every
word that proceeds from the mouth of God.

MATTHEW 4:4

ONE GOOD WAY TO BECOME CENTERED BEFORE stepping onto mealtime's center stage is to recall your deep spiritual connection. While food sustains you, it is only one aspect by which you gain sustenance and strength for your worldly journey. How did Jesus maintain the strength to survive in the wilderness for forty days and nights without food? Clearly, he gained spiritual strength by focusing on prayer and the word of God.

Spiritual energy is a necessary component of fasting. It can also help you overcome other difficult obstacles and challenges. Spiritual focus requires energy and discipline and is like any skill. That is why, in order for you to succeed with any healthy eating plan, you need to engage skillpower, not willpower.

◆

Use the skillpower of spiritual energy
(a prayer, a mindful moment) to help center
yourself before your meal.

Choices

*Man does not live by bread alone. Every now
and then he needs a cookie.*

GROUCHO MARX

IF YOU TAKE YOUR FOOD JOURNEY TOO SERI-
OUSLY, then you will miss out on all the fun and enjoyment and nurturing that food offers you. Moderation means that
you allow yourself the freedom to break rigid boundaries and definitions.

There was a time, for example, when I could not eat just one
cookie. I wanted (maybe "needed") the whole box. One scoop of
ice cream was not adequate. I wanted the whole pint. Today, I can
eat one cookie and be satisfied. Ice cream often remains in the
freezer so long that it has to be tossed out.

When you rigidly set unreasonable standards – zero sugar or
carbs, for example – then who are you punishing and why? Freedom
to choose is not indiscriminate. It comes with the responsibility to
choose wisely. Once you gain strength through skillpower, you will
not have to struggle with an inner battle over food.

◆

Reflect on your rigid definitions and create
a definition of moderation.

Preparations

*A Buddhist master once said, "The most
important thing in spiritual practice is food: when
you eat, how you eat, why you eat."*

LAMA SURYA DAS

WHY IS FOOD SUCH A WONDERFUL SPIRITUAL
practice? One reason is that food nourishes your body, spirit,
and mind. But another important answer is that it brings you face
to face with your physical desires. It is symbolic of the relationship
you have with yourself, as well as a microcosm of the relationship
you have with all things.

The struggle with food serves a positive purpose. It helps you
find balance between your physical being on the one hand and your
spiritual nature on the other. This is why the wisdom traditions
recognize that food can be used as a tool to unite your dual nature
as a physical and a spiritual being. This makes sense because food
becomes part of you, part of your sacred spirit the moment you ingest it. For that reason, each moment of preparation is also sacred.

◆

Clean each surface in your kitchen as you
would any precious, sacred item in your life.

Rituals

Food is not a pleasure race, but a
place to find grace.
DONALD ALTMAN

I ADMIT IT: I AM A FAST EATER. I COME FROM A family of fast eaters that could make a platter of food disappear more quickly than magician David Copperfield. But I'm working on it. Fortunately, the power of mindfulness has helped me discover how ritual brings other dimensions of food to life, such as fulfillment and grace.

A mealtime ritual accomplishes four important things. First, it slows you down, giving you a moment of peace by loosening the stimulus-reaction cycle that drives desire and addiction. Second, it reconnects you with the divine purpose of food to sustain your body and consciousness. Third, it brings you into communion with the divine, the earth, and others. Fourth, it can help establish your food discipline. Even if you say a ritual blessing alone, your thoughts and prayer power connect you with others.

◆

Enjoy a desire-free moment as you
say a blessing.

Eating

In all circumstances serenity of mind should be maintained, and conversation should be conducted as never to mar the harmony of the surroundings.

KAKUZO OKAKURA, *The Book of Tea*

IN THE TEA CEREMONY, THERE IS SOMEONE WHO is called the "first guest." This person's responsibility is to ease the flow of conversation and sociability of the occasion. Other guests take part, too, admiring ancient tea kettles and cups that are used in the ceremony. Everyone who is present recognizes the care and effort that has gone into preserving these timeless antiques and preparing a beautiful tea room with a theme appropriate to the celebration. The result is a sense of wholeness.

Can you hope to accomplish this same sublime process in your home or at any meal? The next time you are a guest, take time to look around. Appreciate the effort and surroundings of your host. Let your words and actions facilitate a sense of oneness and harmony.

◆

Be like the "first guest" at your next meal.

Community

If you want others to be happy, practice compassion.
If you want to be happy, practice compassion.

DALAI LAMA

MUCH FOOD-RELATED UNHAPPINESS COMES from not accepting the way things are. This plays out in many ways: "Why can't I look as good as him/her?" "Why can't I lose weight/stay on my diet/wear a size 2?"

If you are stuck in that place, how can you ever hope to find happiness?

You can begin by practicing compassion for yourself and your own suffering. Compassion does not mean sympathy or pity, where you feel superior to another. The word "compassion" comes from the Latin, meaning "together with" (com) "suffering" (passion). This is true empathy that brings you closer to understanding and loving yourself. Then you can more easily accept, understand, and extend compassion to others.

Thus, when you are together with your own food suffering you can bring wisdom to bear on your situation. You can listen to your wise, compassionate voice. And having done this for yourself, you can do it for others – at mealtime and anytime.

◆

Feel empathy with the food suffering
of yourself or another. What would your
wise voice say?

Departure

*It is when we are in transition that we are
most completely alive.*

WILLIAM BRIDGES, *The Way of Transition*

HAVE YOU EVER DRIVEN THROUGH A FAST-FOOD restaurant and eaten in the car so you could save a few extra seconds? Or run from lunch to your next appointment? I once wrote a poem to describe this:

*There goes a man on the go.
A man who knows
Where to go
To get what he wants
So he can get
Where he wants to go.*

Why are we afraid to take a real rest after meals, even for a moment? I believe it is because at some level we may be frightened of transition. Transition represents what is uncertain, unknown, unproductive, unwanted, unable, etc. It offers no immediate destination or purpose. A moment of transition could last for a day, and if for a day, then why not for a month. The horror of it! (I'm kidding.)

Or, transition can be spacious and life-giving. Used like this, we can fill the space between with rest, peace, and repose.

◆

Use transition to recharge your batteries –
creative or otherwise – for what is to come.

Entry

Not-knowing can be the doorway to true knowing.

SANAYA ROMAN, *Spiritual Growth*

WHEN YOU ENTER A RESTAURANT OR EAT AT home, do you have a set idea of how it will turn out? Do you think the experience will be pleasant or that you will stick to your prearranged diet plan? Yet for one reason or another – a menu change or a food temptation – things do not turn out the way you expected? How do you feel afterward?

In one sense, the idea of "not-knowing" can be about having no expectations. The Buddha made the point that if we accept what is already present in our lives, then we will not be disappointed. Yet the moment we set ourselves up with expectations, we also set ourselves up for unhappiness and dissatisfaction.

Not having expectations does not mean that you have no goals, no hopes, no desires for your next meal. But it does mean that you loosen your grip, ever so slightly, on the outcome.

◆

Acknowledge your mealtime
expectations, then let go a little.

Choices

All things are connected. . . . Man did not weave
the web of life; he is merely a strand in it.
Whatever he does to the web, he does to himself.

TED PERRY, *How Can One Sell the Air?*

EVERY DAY, DECISIONS ARE MADE ABOUT WHAT food products to put on the shelves. Yes, a company might pay a lot of money to have its cereal positioned favorably on the shelf. But if no one buys it, that product will soon be replaced.

It sometimes seems like we are too small, too insignificant to really make a difference. But is this really so? Communal actions have created laws requiring nutritional information on food products. In addition, you make your voice heard each time you make a purchase. By learning which foods are good and which are suspect, you can create more positive change.

When I grew up there were no organic or natural food stores. Today, there are several – and some are nationwide organizations. Let your voice be heard by making informed choices for yourself and the earth.

✦

What foods in your diet are "suspect"?
Commit to finding out more.

Preparations

*After the recipe, I take a deep breath, relax, and
recall that I am in God's presence.*

BROTHER RICK CURRY,
The Secrets of Jesuit Breadmaking

IN YOUR JOURNEY OF FOOD, YOU WOULD BE
mistaken if you thought the only transition time was before
and after the meal. There is always time to reflect on what you are
doing. Always time to take a conscious breath. Always time to
make a sacred connection.

In Christian monastic practice, there is something known as
statio. This is often meant to denote the moment between moments,
or the pause between those times when you are doing things. You
can think of it as a mini-transition. You already experience this several times a day, for example, when you are figuring out what to do
next or when you take a momentary break to regroup.

With *statio* you make the pause intentional. Rest in the now moment. Take a single mindful, desire-free breath and recognize that
there is no other time but this.

✦

Awaken to the wonder of *statio*
throughout your day.

Rituals

Our Father (Mother) who art in heaven,
Hallowed be Thy name.
Thy Kingdom come,
Thy will be done, on earth, as it is in heaven.
Give us this day our daily bread.

TRADITIONAL CHRISTIAN GRACE

 HAVE YOU EVER HEARD OR RECITED GRACE SUCH as the one noted above? I have experienced it when visiting friends or staying in Benedictine monasteries. There are many wonderful traditional ritual blessings such as this one that you can find for use in your own home or when you are out at a restaurant. Should you stick with the same one over and over?

How you use any ritual prayer or blessing is really up to you. Personally, I use a blessing that I have created that draws upon several traditions. At the same time, I vary it as the situation changes. When you allow yourself the freedom to try new blessings and phrases, you can bring what is happening in the moment into your prayers.

◆

How spontaneous can you be
with your blessing?

Eating

In that first bite after my three-week fast,
I learned what all condemned prisoners, downed
pilots, and exiles know: that food is life, and that
eating is saying yes to life.

PHILIP ZALESKI AND PAUL KAUFMAN,
Gifts of the Spirit

AT THE OTHER POLARITY OF EATING IS FASTING.
Have you ever fasted or taken a break from food? Often,
in many traditions, fasting and feasting are linked. Taking a break
(or a brake) from eating, gives you a chance to appreciate food's
value even more. And it lets your digestive system rest.

If you are afraid to go without food for an extended period of
time, there could be many reasons, including the experience of dep-
rivation, of not having had enough food. Having food available at
all times might make you feel safe and secure. These are normal
feelings.

If you constantly eat and do not know why, remember that it is
okay to take an occasional break from eating. In fact, you take a break
from eating each night before you "break-fast" in the morning.

◆

Let go a little bit of your fear of not having
enough to eat. Then appreciate each bite by
saying yes to life.

Community

By concentration an acrobat can walk on a rope.
But the concentration required to tread the path
of truth . . . is far greater.

GANDHI, *Vows and Observances*

HOW CAN YOU BRING TRUTH INTO YOUR RELATIONS with others during meals? Has a meal ever been spoiled because your personal truths do not agree with others?

If you or another becomes angry and narrow-minded at a meal, how does it affect your eating style and choices? Do you find that you eat faster or leave the table with a knot in your stomach? Do you angrily take more dessert to soothe your hurt feelings? Competition and anger at mealtime are counterproductive.

You can begin by recognizing your dogmatic attitudes. Then, let go of them a little with each bite. Experience peace at your mealtime by sharing your empathy, not anger and judgment, with another. When you do this, watch how you change your eating style.

Change your feelings to change your eating.

❖

How does narrow-mindedness
affect your eating?

Departure

*Relying on yourself to do the little things – like
cleaning up carefully after the meal, doing chores
gracefully and mindfully, not banging
kettles – helps develop concentration and
makes practice easier.*

ACHAAN CHAH, BUDDHIST MONK

DO YOU CLEAN UP QUIETLY AND MINDFULLY after a meal? Do you sweep the floor with grace? Or do you leave the kitchen untended and the sink full of dishes?

There is no right or wrong way to approach cleanup. There is only experiencing fully the way you leave your kitchen after eating. Whatever you do, see if you can do it mindfully, with your full attention. If you place the dishes in the sink for washing later, place them thoughtfully. Use this cleaning moment to slow down your actions and your thoughts.

Mindful cleaning will do more than reduce the possibility of broken dishes and accidents. In the long run, it offers compassion toward oneself. If you have not used mindful cleaning, give it a try.

◆

Experience mindful cleaning by slowing
down after a meal.

Entry

Hunger is the mother of anarchy.

HERBERT HOOVER

HUNGER CAN VERY QUICKLY ALTER MOODS IN a negative way. Feelings of nervousness, upset, headaches, even bursts of anger are not uncommon.

Many things can affect your hunger. Skipping meals and not getting a good night's sleep are two actions to avoid. In addition, excess sugar, caffeine, and alcohol may result in mood swings and uneven appetite.

When your hunger causes emotions to get out of control, there are some actions you can take. First, take a mindful breath and note how hunger makes you feel.

Next, make a point of eating something (not junk food) as soon as possible. This will be easier if you develop a backup plan. Have some alternative food of your choosing readily available, such as snacks, a sandwich, or a nutrition drink. You can keep this with you – in your car, briefcase, office, and home refrigerator.

◆

Mindfully note the emotions that
go with your hunger.

Choices

The quality, quantity, method of preparation, way
of consuming, the place, the time, etc., all play an
important part in the effect that food has on us.

DR. VINOD VERMA, *Ayurveda for Life*

PICKING THE FOOD YOU LIKE IS IMPORTANT. However, there is also the question of quality. For example, not all food is as fresh as you think. Apples can be stored for months; tomatoes are often picked before they are ripe and then exposed to nitrogen to make them red. So how do you know if the food you are eating is really fresh and pure?

For one thing, you can go to stores where the produce manager can answer these questions for you. You can also shop at farmers markets, which often require vendors to offer food that is locally grown and fresh from the fields. In addition, look at the expiration dates on packaging to find the freshest products.

And try growing fruits and vegetables of your own. Even if you live in an apartment, you can grow fresh peppers in a pot on a windowsill.

◆

Be mindful of food quality today.

Preparations

*If you are uncertain about a food's preparation,
take care before eating it. Even when eating a
healthful or wholesome food, be attentive to the
energy or atmosphere of the place.*

RABBI NILTON BONDER, *The Kabbalah of Food*

HAS FOOD EVER MADE YOU SICK? FOOD THAT IS unclean, not refrigerated properly, or not cooked long enough can cause illness. The point here is not to get paranoid or fearful about your food.

Most food establishments do an excellent job at maintaining cleanliness. My wife, for example, once owned a sushi franchise. I had the opportunity to learn how to make sushi and obtained a food handler's license. The health regulations were quite demanding, and for good reason. For instance, we protected against cross contamination by using one *makisu* (a bamboo mat used to roll sushi) for raw fish and another for vegetables.

When you go to a restaurant or eat at home, pay attention to cleanliness, natural ingredients, and the care that is put into the food.

✦

Become more aware of the atmosphere
of the place where you eat and the purity of
what you eat.

Rituals

He who eats and drinks, but does not
bless the Lord, is a thief.

JEWISH PROVERB

HAVE YOU EVER MADE A MEAL FOR SOMEONE?
Bought a lunch for someone? Then you know what it is like
to be thanked for your kind giving. Saying a ritual blessing of thanks
is very much like that.

The Jewish tradition, for example, is steeped in blessings. There
are blessings for both bread and wine. The purpose of these and
other blessings is to make food holy and to give thanks to the divine.

When you say a blessing over your meal, you enter sacred space.
From this special place, you can extend your blessing to others.
With each bite you can send blessings of loving kindness to those
you know. You can send prayers to those around the world who do
not have enough to eat. You can take a vow to help the hungry.

Let your blessing grow.

◆

Extend your ritual blessings to others.

Eating

When we lose, I eat. When we win, I eat.
I also eat when it's rained out.

TOMMY LASORDA

ARE YOU SOMEONE WHO GRAZES ON FOOD constantly or is always looking for an eating opportunity? For some people, any time is a good time to eat. The first step to changing this or any fixed eating routine is to become more aware of it.

The problem with grazing is that you may forget how often and how much you eat. It never seems like a large portion of food if you just eat a little bit at a time! Another potential problem is that snack food can be filled with many calories but little nutritional value.

Whether or not you are journaling, become aware of when and why you graze. Do you tend to graze when you are bored, lonely, happy, angry, upset, indifferent, or watching TV?

Let yourself feel this emotion the next time you begin grazing. Then, substitute something, such as a piece of fruit or a glass of water. Eat or drink this mindfully for up to three minutes.

◆

Be mindful of grazing and portion
amount in your next meal.

Community

It is in forgiving that we are forgiven.

SAINT FRANCIS OF ASSISI, *A Simple Prayer*

WHAT IS IT LIKE WHEN YOU EAT WITH OTHERS? Is your critical eating voice on overdrive? Do you wince when someone takes (or refuses) a large helping of dessert? Do you become judgmental when someone eats food that you consider unhealthy, politically incorrect, or ecologically unsound? Or do you worry about others judging you?

You can quiet this critical voice just as Jesus did when he decided that compassion and forgiveness were more important than adhering to the traditional food codes practiced in his day. Jesus felt that criticism of how others ate created unholy judgments and distinctions between people sharing the same table.

There is no perfect way of eating. Besides, no one will eat the way you think is best – even if you know they could benefit from healthier eating habits. For these same reasons, you do not need to judge yourself when you make a mistake.

But when you do, forgive . . . yourself and others.

◆

Be mindful of your judgments simply
by noting them.

Departure

*An integral being knows without going, sees
without looking, and accomplishes without doing.*

LAO TZU, TAOIST PHILOSOPHER

HOW EASILY AND QUICKLY DO YOU LET GO OF your emotions around eating? Do you carry the last meal's badly prepared fish, poor customer service, or thoughtless presentation with you? To do this is to hold on to negative, undigested emotions (and to invite indigestion). Fortunately, you can leave your mealtime disappointments behind by practicing mindful equanimity.

What is mindful equanimity? Equanimity means you take mealtime highs and lows with the same peace and calm. It is a calm, spacious state of mind that does not cling to past mealtime events.

Sit or stand as you breathe slowly, into your belly. Do it for a few breaths, and then scan your body to feel for tension. Once you locate the stress point, inhale deeply, imagining the air filling your area of tension with healing relaxation and coolness. As you exhale, feel the tension and negative mealtime memories leave with the breath.

◆

Be mindful of what you cling to after
the meal. Use each breath to let go of past
negative food emotions.

Entry

Patience takes courage.

PEMA CHÖDRÖN, *Comfortable with Uncertainty*

To ENTER A MEAL WITH PATIENCE AND PEACE IS a way of being gentle and kind. How patient are you as you enter mealtime? Are you patient toward yourself? Toward others?

Patience is not easily understood in our culture. If anything, our lifestyle is greatly measured by speed. Think about it: We drive on expressways. We even check out our food in "express lanes." TV meals are ready in minutes, and some takeout pizza restaurants promise "thirty-minute delivery to your door or your money back."

If you are critical and anxious around the time it takes you to get your meal, you may benefit from relaxing and cultivating patience. When all is said and done, what good are those minutes "saved" in the food checkout express lane if you are all uptight and nervous about it?

◆

Recognize your impatience and
take a mindful breath.

Choices

It's an angry fish because it swims against the tide.
If I'm feeling lethargic I eat salmon.

BOY GEORGE, POP SINGER

 WHEN YOU ARE FEELING SICK OR WEAK, WHAT foods do you instinctively seek out? Do you eat a simpler, more pure and wholesome diet? Do you eat less, giving your body a rest from heavy digestion? (While you are at it, make sure you are getting enough sleep.)

Many traditions accept the idea that you take on the energy characteristics of the food you eat. Practitioners of traditional Chinese medicine place great emphasis on the purity and energy of a food. The right foods are believed to build up and sustain your *chi*, or body's energy. Foods with little nutritional value, such as junk food filled with high levels of sugar and refined starches, do not increase your storehouse of *chi*. Worse, they may weaken it, making you susceptible to disease and exhaustion!

Who knows? There may be a good reason why chicken soup is sometimes called "Jewish penicillin." Whatever your choices, consider how the right foods help your body heal and maintain well-being.

◆

Pay attention to foods that give you a
sense of well-being and those that do not.
Add "well-being" foods to your diet.

Preparations

It is imperative for the tenzo *to actively involve himself personally in both the selection and the preparation of the ingredients.*

Soei Yoneda, *Good Food from the Japanese Temple*

The *tenzo*, or cook, of a monastery does not prepare haphazardly. He is mindful of every little detail. Even the amount of food required for a meal is to be calculated to the grain of rice! How involved are you in the meals you prepare at home?

Even if the extent of your preparation is placing a packaged meal in the oven, you can pay attention to the instructions and the ingredients. How closely, for example, do you read the instructions? Do you ever question or wonder about any of the ingredients? How much food do you waste through preparation? It is okay to question, to doubt, to learn more.

The more connected you become to the source of food, the more involved you are in the preparation and, ultimately, the eating.

◆

Take a more active role in preparation
of today's meal by being mindful of every
detail . . . and consequence.

Rituals

*We can eat for our bodies or we can eat for
our souls. Sabbath eating is to delight in our food,
feasting, and not merely eating.*

DONNA SCHAPER, *Sabbath Keeping*

PERHAPS YOU HAVE NOTICED THAT THE WISDOM traditions have several things in common to connect with the divine, such as ritual cleansing and prayer at mealtime. Some, like the Hindu and Indian traditions, focus on the idea of hospitality by putting the emphasis on sharing food during festivities and showing respect to guests.

How do you "eat for your soul"? Do you have a favorite mode for expressing your spirit through food? Even if you live alone, you can show hospitality by giving away leftover food – to a hungry person or the neighborhood critters and pets. Leftover and even spoiled food make for good compost so you can create more food, more abundance.

When you think about it, everything gets recycled sooner or later. You are just recycling mindfully.

✦

Reflect on a new way to "eat for your soul."

Eating

To find the jewel, one must calm the waves;
it is hard to find if one stirs up the water.

MUMON YAMADA ROSHI, ZEN TEACHER

DOES YOUR MIND RESEMBLE A MURKY POOL AT mealtime? Or is it filled with purpose and clarity? And, how can you tell the difference?

A murky mind is mired in confusion about what foods to eat. Or it critically judges the foods you (and others) eat. It could also be a mind filled with conflicting emotions about dieting and rules to follow when eating.

If your mind is murky, do not fret. In Buddhist lore the lotus represents the awakening consciousness of all beings. Like the lotus, our mind evolves through muddy waters until it blossoms into the jewel of clear consciousness.

Calm your mind and you will find greater food clarity. Build concentration and quiet your mind by mentally repeating a single word to yourself during a silent meal. Or just focus on mindful eating through setting an intention for each movement you make.

✦

Find a meaningful word to calm
your mind, such as: Peace, Father,
Mother, Love, God, Jesus, Buddha, One,
Shalom, Om, Salaam.

Community

*From my own personal experience I can tell you
that when I practice altruism and care for others, it
immediately makes me calmer and more secure.*

DALAI LAMA, *Transforming the Mind*

NO MATTER HOW MUCH OF A CHALLENGE YOUR eating or dieting issues are, you are not alone in your pain. And, even if you are at a state of relative peace with your eating, there are ways to lessen the pain of others.

In some traditions, the idea of offering help to others is not voluntary, but necessary and essential. The Jewish experience of *mitzvah*, or good deeds, is a practice by which service to others is commanded by God. Feeding the hungry, inviting others to dinner, and giving charity to the homeless are not optional!

A *mitzvah*, or good deed, is not a burden but a personal bliss. It is a bliss to know that by feeding others you can make a difference. This is empowerment, too, because you help others to sustain themselves and grow as a result.

◆

Discover your *mitzvah* and feel the benefits.

Departure

*Change can happen at any time, but transition comes
along when one chapter of your life is over and
another is waiting in the wings to make its entrance.*

WILLIAM BRIDGES, *The Way of Transition*

THE PREVIOUS MEAL AND WAY OF EATING IS OVER.
The next chapter is yet to be written. How you feel about
the most recently "eaten" chapter is part of the process of letting go.

According to William Bridges, change is simply a situational
shift. It is during the transition where we do all the work. Transition
has three stages: letting go, the neutral zone, and beginning again.

- Letting go can be difficult. Each time you commit to a new
  diet, for example, you must say goodbye to certain foods that
  you enjoy.
- The neutral zone represents chaos and uncertainty – where
  you do not know what will happen next. How will you adapt
  to the new "chapter" of eating, diet, and foods?
- Beginning again is the place where you take hold of that new
  chapter or diet, make it your own, and try it on for size.

Still, change and transition with food are a constant. This is one
book that you never really complete.

◆

What food transition are you
experiencing right now?

Entry

*The Sabbath is a bride, and its celebration
is like a wedding.*

ABRAHAM JOSHUA HESCHEL, *The Sabbath*

DO YOU CELEBRATE YOUR EVERY MEAL? DO YOU ever imagine that you could? Well, you can. Just use your entry time to explore your options and get a sense of the joy that your next meal offers.

How about: Eating at an outdoor café or park? Laughing and sharing stories with friends and associates? Sitting in sublime, quiet solitude? Eating while reading a favorite book or watching a favorite TV talk show host?

Use your entry moment to tap into and express your creativity. Making each meal a celebration means that you honor that meal, just as you honor someone's birthday, graduation, or anniversary. Put a new celebratory spin on your eating and let go of the burden.

By adding new meaning to your meal or diet, you are also honoring yourself and creating a new relationship to food.

◆

How can I honor today's meal?

Choices

Feed the sacred flame with healthy food at
proper intervals . . . for the maintenance of
a robust and healthy body.

GOPI KRISHNA, *Kundalini*

HOW HAS YOUR WINTER DIET PREPARED YOU FOR the coming of spring? If you live in a snowy winter climate, do you eat a lot of warm, heavy dishes that fortify you against the cold? If you live in a warm winter locale, how does your eating change with the seasons?

Is your eating in tune with the new season? Spring is only officially a day away, but the signs of it are already evident. Slowly but surely the days are lengthening. The rains of March and April prepare the ground for planting. The trees awaken with buds.

Do you feel yourself awakening to the call of lighter, cooler, fresher foods? Are you feeling more energetic as the days lengthen? What foods are grown in your regional area? You might want to try them, even if you never have.

◆

Feel the seasonal change of the food
your body needs.

Preparations

*Life is not hurrying on to a receding future, nor
hankering after the imagined past. It is the turning
aside like Moses to the miracle of the lit bush.*

CELTIC PRAYER

THE VERNAL EQUINOX OCCURS ON OR AROUND
this date, and it marks the beginning cycle of the new seasonal year. With this new cycle come new hope, growth, life, activity, possibility, transformation, and vitality.

What new seasonal shift or transformation can you introduce into your daily preparation? Maybe you can make a shift in emotional attachment, such as letting go of negative emotions around food and eating. Or perhaps you can prepare your table and dining space in a way that is in harmony with the ideals of growth and hope. In addition, your new cycle of preparation could explore the possibility of crafting a meal that combines both winter and spring foods.

As the days lengthen and you become more active, follow suit by integrating mindful walking or exercising into your preparation.

◆

Bring fresh "spring" energy to
your preparation.

Rituals

For the more prayer is received, rather than made,
the more genuine it will be.

THELMA HALL, *Too Deep for Words*

DOES YOUR RITUAL BLESSING RECEIVE IN THE deepest sense? This question asks you to think about the difference between making a prayer and receiving one. Realize that this subtle distinction can have a real impact on how you eat and feel about your meal.

Your ritual blessing sets the stage for what follows. For example, if you make a blessing, then you are proactive and being in charge – just as when you take food. Taking in this fashion is often based on your physical needs, craving, and desires.

On the other hand, when you receive a blessing, then you tap into a bigger process. You offer yourself up to the mercy and grace of the divine. You accept what is given with a great and open heart. It follows, then, that you open yourself to receiving food in this same way – letting it come to you without greed, desire, and hunger.

Shift your blessing toward receiving and you can slowly but surely shift your eating from emotional hunger and greed to sacred eating and accepting. You can take food, or you can receive it.

◆

Sit in spacious silence. Open yourself to
receiving a mealtime blessing. Whatever you
experience is your blessing.

Eating

Next time you're in a buffet or cafeteria line,
notice how some people behave.

RONA KABATZNICK, PH.D., *The Zen of Eating*

HAVE YOU EVER BEEN TO AN ALL-YOU-CAN-EAT buffet? One exercise I often suggest to participants in my Mindful and Sacred Eating Workshops is to visit an all-you-can-eat buffet or fast-food restaurant. Then, just observe. I ask the observers to pretend that they are visiting from another planet and have absolutely no idea what food and eating is all about. Then, just watch (unobtrusively, of course) without judgment, craving, or opinion. (If you try this, eat beforehand so you are neither tempted nor repulsed!)

Often, eating taps into your fear of not getting enough food, abundance, health, success, love, protection, etc. An all-you-can-eat buffet offers a kind of food security blanket. It seems to say, "You will be taken care of. You will have enough." And so the tendency is to eat as much as possible and hedge against future scarcity.

If you watch this enactment without judgment, you can experience deep compassion for the underlying pain and suffering that causes eating from a place of fear and need for security and well-being.

◆

Experience compassion for how you
(and others) eat.

Community

*The tree has its own pace. Your job is to
dig a hole, water and fertilize it, and protect it
from insects. . . . But the way the tree grows
is up to the tree.*

ACHAAN CHAH, BUDDHIST MONK

DO YOU FIND THAT YOUR FOOD STRUGGLES make it difficult for you to eat with others? This is not uncommon. But in fact, one possible way to help heal your own food issue may be to use food altruistically in a communal setting.

I know one young woman, for example, who struggled with disordered eating. She feared food, restricted her intake, and rarely ate with others. By practicing mindfulness over a period of time, she relaxed to the point where she invited a couple to her home for dinner. She experienced a breakthrough after sharing food with others. This communal meal helped her experience food for what it can give to others. It put her on the solution side of food instead of the problem side.

If and when you are ready to do this, focus on the giving of food to others. Start slow by inviting one or two close friends. Share and experience the nourishment of goodwill and love at mealtime.

◆

Reflect on planting new seeds
in your diet and life.

Departure

The true purpose of exercise is to invigorate and
strengthen us in body, mind, and spirit.
DEEPAK CHOPRA, *Overcoming Addictions*

IF YOU DRIVE TO A RESTAURANT, DO YOU ALWAYS try to find the closest parking spot? Believe it or not, parking farther away and walking could lead to changing how and what you eat.

I know of a woman who could not stop smoking. She tried everything from the nicotine patch to hypnosis. Nothing worked until she started exercising. As soon as she realized smoking was incompatible with her new lifestyle, she easily "let go" of the habit with no struggle! This story offers hope for anyone struggling with food and dieting.

To change any habit takes skill and practice. It is easier to drop a habit if you replace it with a more skillful, enjoyable, and beneficial one. Start where you are. Even a twenty-second stroll is a good place to start.

✦

Add a new skillful lifestyle habit (exercise,
sport, walking) to complement your meal.

Entry

Ask and it will be given to you; seek and you will
find; knock and the door will be opened to you.

LUKE 11:9

IS THERE A DEEPER SPIRITUAL MEANING OR message you would like to receive at mealtime? By entering into prayer even before eating, you can be more ready to receive the inner nourishment and fulfillment of food, rather than just getting filled up. Jesus' teaching on prayer is not confined to the blessing portion of your meal. In truth, prayer extends beyond mealtime.

You can get the most out of your meal by centering and becoming mindful in advance. Sometimes, reading something sacred, poetic, or meaningful can help.

Do you have a favorite passage from scripture or a book? Spend a few moments and read a short passage (three or four paragraphs) over and over. Do not try to impose any meaning. Just steep yourself in the words for a few minutes and see how it changes your mindfulness as you prepare to eat.

◆

Prepare to enter your meal mindfully
and centered by reading something
special in advance.

Choices

*Other guests are slower to arrive. The banquet is
almost over; they are served only leftovers.*

Sara Sviri, *The Taste of Hidden Things*

 Have you ever eaten the same food so often
that you do not really taste it? When this happens, or when
you are distracted, you are not arriving at your own meal, your own
banquet. You eat, but you do not taste.

In the Sufi tradition, an experience (especially a mystical one) is
appropriately called a "taste." One Sufi story tells of guests who arrive on time to partake of a most incredible banquet. But those
who arrive late miss their taste because the food is already gone.
Are you missing out on your taste because you narrow your choices
until only a few foods remain at the banquet? Or perhaps you do
not fully taste your food?

Practice this: Take a single raisin, olive, or peanut and spend
three entire minutes eating it. Chew each small bite until it becomes liquid in your mouth. Experience the whole taste.

◆

Mindfully spend three minutes (or longer)
eating a raisin, nut, or olive.

Preparations

*Maintain an attitude that tries to build great
temples from ordinary greens.*

DOGEN, THIRTEENTH-CENTURY ZEN MASTER

 WHAT HAPPENS WHEN YOU SLAP TOGETHER A meal? Do you ever later think about that little extra touch that would have made that sandwich (salad, soup, dessert) special?

The preparation stage lets you make even simple food exceptional, as Zen master Dogen advises. First, visualize what you hope to create. In your mind's eye, imagine the meal's scent, look, and taste. Then, be the architect of that "temple" by going beyond your normal methods, routines, and recipes.

Presentation is another key ingredient. Whether you eat alone or with others, you can appreciate the artistry and effort that goes into your meal. And even if your meal comes in a prepackaged container, you can arrange the contents on plates along with other foods.

◆

Turn your ordinary meal into
something special with skillful presentation
and preparation.

Rituals

*When you have total intention to create
something . . . it simply cannot fail to manifest.*
SHAKTI GAWAIN, *Creative Visualization*

WITH RITUAL, YOU CAN CREATE AND USE AN IN-
tention that specifically states your daily commitment to
eat a better diet, achieve health, and lose excess weight, etc. In this
way, your ritual blessing serves a practical purpose – to actualize
your deepest hopes and desires through intention. (If you want,
your intention can extend beyond mealtime issues and into other
areas of your life.)

First, make a commitment to say a ritual before each meal. Then,
you will want to follow what Shakti Gawain describes as the following three steps: "You deeply desire it, you completely believe
that you can do it, and you are totally willing to have it."

To help you stay disciplined, repeat your intention at each meal.
But you still need to be skillful in your choices for the long term.
If you stumble from cheesecake to cheesecake and never exercise,
the intention of being thinner and healthy will not be enough to
materialize a healthy body.

◆

Create a practical blessing with your total
intention, then follow up with skillful action.

Eating

*The more you experience yourself as energy,
the easier it is not to identify yourself
with your physical body.*

ANDREW WEIL, *Spontaneous Healing*

DO YOU IDENTIFY MORE STRONGLY WITH YOUR physical body or your "energy" body? Each approach affects how you eat and the emotions you feel around eating.

If you worry a lot about how your body looks, fret over dress or pants size, and always think about how much (or little) you eat, then you identify with the physical body. Do you see how this approach is outward-focused? In addition, it is difficult to hold the physical body up to an ideal because it is always changing and aging.

But if you experience yourself as energy, then you will be concerned with getting enough aerobic exercise and eating food that nourishes you with uplifting energy. Food's purpose shifts to the longevity and health of your energy body. This is because the energy body manifests and maintains the physical body.

So while good energy food will help your physical body – only you can let go of some of the worry.

◆

Eat today's meal for your energy body.

Community

*Your Sangha – family, friends, and
co-practitioners – is the soil, and you are the seed.*

THICH NHAT HANH, *Cultivating the Mind of Love*

DO THOSE AROUND YOU SUPPORT YOUR EFFORT
to eat a better diet? In Buddhism, the Sangha represents a
community of like-minded persons seeking the truth. Members
are supportive of each other's pursuits.

When it comes to food, though, everyone has a different idea
of what is right, best, healthy, etc. There may be times when a partner, friend, or family member will not understand why you want to
change eating habits. (Change can be scary for others, too.) At
times, they may even tempt you with exactly the food you do not
want to eat!

The Buddha said that whom we associate with is very important.
Even if you cannot change an association, find social support from
others who are trying just as you are. Find a friend who you can
call when you need someone to champion your efforts.

◆

Have a meal with someone who supports
your healthy eating efforts.

Departure

The winner sows hatred because the loser suffers.
Let go of winning and losing and find joy.

THE BUDDHA, *Dhammapada*

DO YOU EVER COMPARE YOUR EATING WITH others? Do you ever think, "I'm eating healthier (or worse) than he is." "Why don't I have willpower like her?" "How can they eat those foods and not gain weight?"

Eating is not a competition. If you measure your own eating habits against others, then you will feel superior, inferior, happy, or regretful, depending on how you stack up. But the feeling is only temporary. You have to start comparing all over again at the next meal. Is it really worth it?

Without comparison there is no winner, no loser, and no striving to change the moment. There is acceptance of your eating and tolerance of others' eating. There is just mindfulness: this food, you eating, chewing and swallowing, and you receiving nourishment.

◆

Acknowledge comparison and rest in
mindfulness at your meal.

Entry

*My doctor told me to stop having intimate dinners
for four. Unless there are three other people.*
ORSON WELLES

A STRONG APPETITE CAN DRIVE YOU TO DISTRAC-
tion. Prior to a meal, has your appetite ever caused you to
buy more in a grocery store or order more in a restaurant than you
(or maybe Orson Welles) could eat at one sitting? If so, welcome
to the club.

Having a good appetite is important because it means you feel
your body and its needs. Appetite is useful for another reason. It can
help you more deeply tune into your hunger.

Have you ever tried to distinguish between three different kinds
of appetite? First, there is your hunger that is provoked by sense
desire (seeing, tasting, touching, or smelling food). Next, there is appetite that is stimulated by your physical need for energy or nourishment, and your body's internal clock. Lastly, there is craving for
food that is provoked by habit or emotional conditioning, such as
wanting comfort food when feeling stressed or lonely.

◆

Awaken to the deeper cause
of today's appetite.

Choices

*People are capable of tremendous self-sacrifice and
self-giving when they are in love. . . . The center of
the person's life has become the beloved.*

THELMA HALL, *Too Deep for Words*

 HAVE YOU EVER BEEN TOO ILL OR SICK TO EAT?
When you felt better, did you choose that first meal carefully – as you might for a beloved (yourself)?

If you are going to choose foods that are truly life-sustaining and enhancing, then you need to feel like the most precious beloved one in your life! Before eating, you can practice loving kindness toward yourself.

Find a quiet and peaceful place. Sit with your eyes closed, and imagine yourself as a young child (or adult) worthy of love. Then, envision a caring benefactor (a parent, ancestor, or spiritual friend) who sends you a deep wish for your total well-being and happiness.

Let this heartfelt wish flow into your heart. Even if this takes time, stay with it until you feel love flowing through your whole body. Then repeat over and over: "From this space of love may I choose the foods that offer me health and well-being."

◆

Practice loving kindness toward yourself
for five to ten minutes before choosing
what you will eat.

Preparations

Be prepared.

Boy Scout motto

 Did you ever experience how the lack of preparation could drastically alter a meal? Lacking a simple utensil, like a corkscrew or can opener, might mean missing out on something special. Improvising can be fun, but it is always nice to have all the choices available to you.

Cooking and preparing a meal is a lot like going camping. If you forget to bring along your flashlight, you might have a difficult time putting up the tent. That is why mealtime preparation is for your own benefit and peace of mind.

Appreciate the beauty, precision, and effort that went into crafting each utensil and tool. Clean and care for these tools as you would a precious instrument or jewel. The right tools can truly help make your meal blissful, sacred, and memorable.

◆

Appreciate how the right utensils complete
the sacredness of preparation.

Rituals

*The Indians addressed all of life as a "thou" – the
trees, the stones, everything. You can address
anything as a "thou," and if you do it, you can feel
the change in your own psychology.*

JOSEPH CAMPBELL, *The Power of Myth*

DID YOU EVER SPEND TIME IN THE COUNTRY
or on a farm witnessing the lives of farmers, animals, plants,
and the food closer up? A ritual act can serve the same purpose of
bringing you into contact with both the source of food and what
Joseph Campbell refers to as "thou."

When I was in my twenties, for example, I awakened to my de-
pendence on the growers of food and plant and animal life. At that
time I spent a couple of days on a family-run Wisconsin dairy farm,
witnessing up close the relationship between the dairy farmer and
the cows that provide the milk and cheese products I had taken
for granted. I got a sense of how the land had been cared for and
worked by this family through several generations.

The next time you say a blessing of gratitude over your food,
know that the taste it contains touches more than you can imagine.

◆

Experience the sacred "thou" as you
invoke your ritual blessing.

Eating

Dieting is murder on the road. Show me a man
who travels and I'll show you one who eats.

BRUCE FROEMMING, BASEBALL UMPIRE

ARE THERE TIMES WHEN YOU FIND IT ESPECIALLY difficult to eat mindfully and with awareness? For some, traveling can trigger mindless eating and craving. For others, any tense situation that takes you out of your comfort zone can cause this. What takes you from mindful to mindless eating?

It is easier to manage food and mindfulness when you are in your own environment and emotionally calm. The trick is to be able to bring mindfulness with you – regardless of the stresses and location where you happen to be.

Whenever you feel vulnerable to mindless eating, take a mindful breath between each bite. Then, count the number of times that you chew. Together, these two mindful simple practices will slow you down and bring you back to mindfulness.

◆

Invite mindful eating with awareness
of breath and chewing.

Community

*If you sat for fifteen minutes repeating
"hate, hate, hate," you would be the worse for it;
yet this is just what we do when we keep
dwelling on resentments.*

EKNATH EASWARAN, *The Mantram Handbook*

HAVE YOUR EVER DIRECTED THE REFRAIN "BLAME, blame, blame," or "shame, shame, shame," or "should have, should have, should have," at yourself or others during a meal? Instead of dwelling on what you think or feel is wrong, you can use food and community to catapult you into a positive state of mind and emotions.

The great Hindu sage Vivekananda felt that most people too readily focus on their personal weaknesses instead of their vast heritage of knowledge and wholeness. I believe you can tap into this wholeness simply by reciting positive thoughts during your meal. You can, for example, silently repeat a word or phrase such as "love," "loving kindness," or "living kindness" over and over.

Even in response to negative energy or comments from others, you can repeat your phrase to keep you from reacting – and actually affect others. As you do so, do not forget to feel the love that is also in the food you chew.

◆

Send love to others during your meal.

Departure

*The lunches of fifty-seven years had caused his
chest to slip down to the mezzanine floor.*

P. G. WODEHOUSE

DO YOU FEEL LIKE YOUR BODY HAS SHIFTED IN new directions after you eat – maybe even toward the mezzanine? Or do you feel light, awake, and invigorated? It pays to take notice of your mealtime departure.

What does it feel like to eat a little less (or more) than you are used to eating? Do you feel uncomfortable or unsatisfied? Departure time is a good time to notice how much you need to feel full. Also, take time to sense how fulfilling the meal has been to you at this time. If you do not feel physically and mentally well, then maybe a change of diet is in order.

You can even add to your fulfillment after the meal. Take a stroll. Sit outside for a moment. Have a pleasant conversation with someone. Note something pleasant in your life at this very moment.

◆

Feel your body after mealtime and
note something pleasant.

Entry

*True healing begins with awareness: awareness
of self, first of all, to discover how we function.
With awareness comes responsibility.*

ANNEMARIE COLBIN, *Food and Healing*

DO YOUR BODY AND MIND SPEAK THE SAME LAN-
guage before mealtime? Are they like the proverbial Venus
and Mars, misunderstanding one another although they cannot
live apart? Which one is more in control and determines your eating style?

When your mind is in control, you may seek food to medicate,
or feed, your emotional feelings such as boredom, emptiness, escape, the need for love, etc. These emotional states can manifest in
many ways. Many new mothers, for example, have told me that the
effort of feeding and nurturing their newborns leaves them emotionally depleted and in need of nurturing – which is often done with
food.

Conversely, your body might control your eating if you are very
sensitive and reactive. When your stomach grumbles or you feel
heartburn, do you automatically assume you need to eat? Or have
you trained your body to eat at certain times throughout the day?

◆

Why are you hungry? Today,
be aware of your emotional hunger
and your body hunger.

Choices

I went to a restaurant. It said "Breakfast anytime."
So I ordered French toast during the Renaissance.

STEVEN WRIGHT, COMEDIAN

DO YOU EVER FEEL LIKE YOU ARE MISSING OUT on the bliss and fun of food? Choosing foods is not supposed to be drudgery. Strict diet plans and food struggles, however, can make this process end up feeling clinical and forced. You were born to eat food naturally and intuitively. So how can you slowly but surely return to feeding your natural body with natural mindfulness and natural food selection?

Natural food selection implies that you are in balance. This means that you naturally select a variety of foods to meet the needs of your physical and energy body – which includes your consciousness. The first step in natural, balanced eating is to recognize if you are in balance! You probably know the answer to this if you eat for emotional reasons, have trouble eating in moderation (too much or too little), or constantly think and worry about food.

Before making today's food choices, imagine this: If foods were your friends, which ones would you want over for your meal? Think intuitively about how you would feel after visiting with these "friends."

◆

Let intuition guide you to one new
choice for today's meal.

Preparations

The most indispensable ingredient of all good
home cooking: love for those you are cooking for.

Sophia Loren

Can you recall any memorable meals from childhood? Do you remember a special holiday time you had with those you cared about? Such is the power of food cooked with love.

Personally, for example, I can still feel the love from those Sundays I spent at my grandparent's apartment in Chicago. My extended family was present, including cousins and often a new guest from out of town. But what really made the day special was the food my grandmother prepared from scratch. Her freshly baked apple pie and exotic eastern European foods – such as gefilte fish and matzo ball soup – were the highlight of the night. I am certain the love my grandmother had for us went into that food.

How do you approach preparation and cooking? Think about those you are cooking for with love, and your whole meal can be infused with a sense of bliss, joyousness, and wholeness.

✦

Prepare a meal or snack for yourself
(and others) with love.

Rituals

To develop a disciplined way of life, you need to
look at your own situation.... At this point
you are your own witness.

KALU RINPOCHE, *The Dharma*

RITUALS CAN SERVE MANY PURPOSES. THEY CAN put you in touch with spirit, break patterns by slowing you down, and even help you gain discipline and strength at mealtime.

There is a wonderful metaphor, used by Kalu Rinpoche and others, about two houses, each containing a treasure. One house has only one door that is locked shut. The other house has an unlocked door and all the windows are open. It is not hard to imagine which house will have its treasure stolen!

How well do you guard your true treasure – your one and only body? With ritual, you can. There is a Buddhist precept, for example, that asks the practitioner to refrain from taking any substance (food, drink, drugs) that could affect mindfulness. Each tradition has something you can use with a ritual to guard against mindless eating. Use what speaks to you.

❖

With your ritual blessing, add a precept or
vow of mindful discipline at today's meal.

Eating

Money is only one example of a system
that weaves Enchantment . . . and we end up
believing that the picture the system presents
us is what life actually is.

KEN MCLEOD, *Wake Up to Your Life*

FOOD, LIKE MONEY, CAN REPRESENT A SYSTEM that weaves enchantment. Sometimes we buy into a food system and think that it is the answer. I am not saying that you should not eat a particular diet if it makes you feel healthy and energetic. However, when you make food your goal, not your process, it can affect you and others.

For example, Buddha ate meat when it was offered to him. Yet Hitler was a vegetarian. Think of it this way: Would you rather have as your neighbor a kind meat eater or a cruel vegetarian? The truth is that none of us fit into neat little packages.

Dr. Steven Bratman even coined a term – orthorexia nervosa – to describe an obsession with eating healthy. Any system of eating that becomes obsessive can limit your view.

◆

Ask yourself: What is my food system?
Am I obsessive about it to my or
another's detriment?

Community

We may in fact disappoint ourselves, may not
meet our own expectations, but we do not cease to
be a friend to ourselves.

SHARON SALZBERG, *Loving-Kindness*

HAVE YOU EVER FELT ANY DISAPPOINTMENT around food? Have you disappointed yourself by not keeping your word about a diet? Have you ever disregarded the advice of a nutritionist or doctor? Have you ever felt disgust or dismay at the diet of someone who you think eats too much or too little?

You can reduce disappointment at mealtime by practicing a kind of friendship that is universal. Loving-kindness friendship means you feel a deep wish for the well-being and happiness of another, regardless of whether you know them. This kind of love is not sentimental, nostalgic, or physical. As such, it cannot cause us to feel jealousy and envy and loss.

Where does loving kindness begin? By loving yourself first. As a friend, forgive yourself your disappointments and your expectations.

◆

Be your own friend and forgive
your disappointments while eating
with others (or alone).

Departure

*By becoming a conscious choice-maker, you
begin to generate actions that are evolutionary for
you and for those that are around you. And that's
all you need to do.*

DEEPAK CHOPRA, *The Seven Spiritual Laws of Success*

AS A CONSCIOUS CHOICE MAKER, YOU CAN DECIDE to leave behind the emotions from the meal you just ate. This one action will have many consequences. By letting go of your mealtime emotions, you free up your emotional range to whatever is present in this new moment.

Suppose you are unhappy with your meal choices. If you carry this with you, you may feel depressed and guilty. In this state of mind you may decide to isolate yourself instead of being with others and engaging in life. Or, your emotions may cause you to feel like you need to comfort yourself – so you end up eating more and feeling even worse.

We make thousands and thousands of lifetime choices. Become just a little more aware of your emotional choices and you will create new actions that could change your day in surprising ways.

◆

Choose to leave food emotions
at your meal and open to whatever
the new moment brings.

Entry

*Knowledge of what is possible is
the beginning of happiness.*

GEORGE SANTAYANA, PHILOSOPHER

SUPPOSE YOU KNEW THAT YOUR NEXT MEAL would be the most amazing and profound experience of your life? How would that change your next meal? Frankly, you would probably run there as fast as you could.

As strange as it may sound, your next meal can be the beginning of happiness. It can be the dawn of greater awareness of your food habits. It can be the awakening of a food memory. It can be the first time you make a new food choice. It can present a new way of communing with the divine. It can be a window into making a deeper connection with someone. It can even offer you a mindful taste and a new flavor of food.

All this, and more, is possible. It is all waiting for you . . . at your next meal.

◆

Be aware of what is possible as you
enter your next meal.

Choices

Choices focus our lives. They monogram our
towels. They sign our name to our life.

DONNA SCHAPER, *Sabbath Keeping*

 IN GENERAL, DO YOU SOMETIMES FEEL THAT THE number of choices you have to make is overwhelming? In this context, food is just another decision that has to be made. So, while choices can be fun, they can be understandably difficult, too.

The number of choices you make on a daily basis is staggering. Just in the morning, for instance, you must decide when to set your alarm clock and wake up. Because you are pressed for time, you may limit your morning choices and settle into an automatic routine that gets ready to greet the day. On top of that, you must decide if you are hungry and what you might want to eat for breakfast. Unfortunately, the morning breakfast often becomes a victim to routine as well.

No wonder it is easy to take a habitual path to eating. Habit reduces choices and lets you eat what is familiar, with few surprises.

♦

Be aware of how your routine affects
your appetite and shapes what you eat in the
morning. Is your habit beneficial?

Preparations

*If a man has never been pleasantly surprised at
the way custard sets or flour thickens, there is not
much hope of making a cook of him.*

ROBERT FARRAR CAPON, AUTHOR

IN MANY WAYS, MINDFULNESS DURING PREPA-
ration is like the ancient practice of alchemy – it transforms
one element into another that is even more precious. As you prepare any meal, you can use mindfulness to set a pace and attention
to sensation that carries over into all of your eating experiences
and themes.

Place your focus on the handling of food. Even if you are taking
a frozen dinner out of the freezer, feel the coolness of the carton
on your skin. Examine the texture of the food you prepare. Is it
soft, hard, grainy, fuzzy? Is it wet, moist, or dry? What about the
color?

As you experience these sensations, listen to your mind's reaction. Do you find each sensation to be pleasant, unpleasant, or neutral? When your mind skips ahead to something else, gently bring
it back to the sensation.

◆

Be mindful of sensations as you
prepare a meal.

Rituals

*May the Lord accept this, our offering, and bless
our food that it may bring us strength in our body,
vigor in our mind, and selfless devotion in our
heart for His service.*

PARAMANDA, HINDU SAGE

USING DEVOTION IN A MEALTIME RITUAL IS A powerful and engaging experience. With it, you can experience blessing, gratitude, and selflessness at the same time. One aspect of devotional prayer is receiving and sending your love to God.

A devotional ritual like the one by Paramanda opens up your heart, not only to the divine, but to all things you find at your mealtime. If you are not particularly religious, you can think of devotional practice as opening you up to the mystery of nature and the Earth, or your devotion to your family. This is your opportunity to express in words how you feel in your heart.

You can even create your own devotional ritual by writing down how you connect with the divine source. Adapt from other prayers, poems, or make this devotion uniquely yours.

◆

Express your deepest heart connection
with the divine over your meal.

Eating

There's only one secret to bachelor cooking –
not caring how it tastes.

P. J. O'ROURKE, AMERICAN HUMORIST AND JOURNALIST

BACHELORS SOMETIMES DO NOT KNOW ANY BETTER. I can remember living with a roommate when I was a college junior. Having had very little experience in preparation and cooking, however, our meals were often tasteless, or worse. Yet I could accept this because food was not the most important thing in my life at that time.

Your attitude about a food (and life) can greatly affect how it tastes on a particular day. If you are very restrictive of what you eat on account of taste, you might focus on taste just as bare sensation. This may help you add some new foods to your diet.

Have you ever described the flavor of food – much as a scientist might – without being attached to how much you liked or disliked it? One secret of mindful eating is to just taste the bare sensation without opinion. See if taste changes as you chew the food. How does the location of food on your tongue affect the taste? You may discover, for example, that food you like (or dislike) tastes different when you remove the attitude and just taste it without the emotion.

◆

Be a scientist and just taste the taste
of food as you eat. Note your likes and
dislike, but stay focused on taste.

Community

It isn't so much what's on the table
that matters, as what's on the chairs.

W. S. GILBERT, PLAYWRIGHT

WHEN YOU SHARE A POTLUCK MEAL WITH FRIENDS, family, and associate, what do you usually remember the most? Is it the food? The companionship? Or a combination of both?

Buddha often made the point that those you choose to be around greatly impact your life. This is very true at mealtime as well. Whom you are with can change your dietary plans, your approach to eating, and how you feel about the entire get-together.

If you are struggling with food, become aware of how the people you eat with affect your own eating and choices. Do you tend to eat mindlessly or become emotionally upset, for example, when you eat in the company of people who are critical of your eating?

When you find yourself becoming upset or mindless in your eating, take a mindful breath and return to the peace of this precious moment.

◆

Think about how your guests
affect your food struggle.

Departure

With each inhalation, your body takes in tens of
billions of atoms, tiny fragments of the universe
that over the centuries have passed through
countless numbers of other living beings and will
continue to do so long after you are no longer here.

DEEPAK CHOPRA, *Overcoming Addiction*

 AT THE MOST BASIC LEVEL, FOOD PASSES THROUGH you, charging you up like a battery. Then, it is gone, leaving no traces behind or being miraculously transformed into cells in your body.

As you depart your meal, know that food is doing what it is supposed to do. Its primary purpose is, after all, to nourish you. It is not an enemy whose purpose is to make you grow fat, unattractive, and undesirable. Neither is it a friend that will make you pretty, handsome, and svelte.

If you emphasize choices that enhance the nourishment and well-being of your energy body, then you can let the meal go. But if your emotions are tied into how your body looks, then letting go may be more difficult.

✦

After your meal, focus on your energy body
and let go of mealtime emotions.

Entry

I always plan dinner first thing in the morning.
That's the only way I can get through the day,
having a specific meal to look forward to at night.

ALAN KING

DO YOU EVER PLAN A MEAL FAR IN ADVANCE? When you are done with breakfast, for example, are you already thinking about what to eat for lunch? If so, then food is obviously very important in your life. But too much preoccupation with planning food and meals can lead to an addictive or obsessive attitude.

If you are on a diet or restricting food of any kind, then this may be a reason why you think a lot about food. This could mean you are not getting enough to eat. I know of one man who narrowed his food choices to a few vegetables a day. He was fighting hunger constantly, and often binged late at night – usually on bread and other foods that his body craved. Sometimes cravings are for a good reason. If you are on a diet and have food cravings or think about food all the time, talk with a health professional.

◆

Become aware of your cravings
when dieting.

Choices

Surrender is choice – an absolute, personal choice.

EMMANUEL, *Emmanuel's Book*

 HAVE YOU EVER SURRENDERED TO THE TEMPTATION for drink or food? Welcome to the human race. If you blame yourself for giving in, that is not much of a surprise. In our culture, to surrender is often associated with losing. In truth, surrendering to food means you give in to an indulgence with mindful awareness, rather than blame or guilt. This mindful surrender helps loosen – ever so slightly – the automatic cycle of stimulus and reaction.

Sometimes you may confuse surrender with submission. When you submit to something, you have no choice, no freedom, and no will. If you force yourself to submit to a diet, for example, you may ignore the signals and signs in your body that tell you to change course. To surrender is different.

Mindful surrender leaves you in charge. With mindfulness, you can surrender to your body's craving with compassion. Good news: Mindful surrender strengthens you the next time you face a similar choice.

◆

Surrender mindfully today when
your body needs to eat.

Preparations

Sunbeams may be extracted from cucumbers.

SENATOR DAVID DAGGET,
NINETEENTH-CENTURY U.S. SENATOR

HAVE YOU ANY EXPERIENCE SLICING AND DICING vegetables? It takes a lot of time. If you have ever made sushi, a salad, or snacks, then you know that the experience of simple preparation can be either tedious or blissful. The choice is yours, and mindfulness makes all the difference in the world.

First, do not rush the job. That is when more than the cucumber gets sliced! Allow yourself enough time to prepare in a way that lets you mindfully enjoy the process. Clean your workspace. Then, gather and arrange all your foods and utensils before you begin.

You can also give more meaning to your preparation by setting the intention not to waste any food – such as by composting. Your preparation could include the intention of giving additional food to those who may need it – even if it is the neighborhood critters.

◆

Slow down and extract sunbeams
from today's preparation.

Rituals

*Eat your bread with joy, drink your wine
with a merry heart.*

ECCLESIASTES 9:7

YOU CAN THINK OF A MEALTIME RITUAL AS ANOTHER
table setting – an additional guest who brings a heaping of
wisdom, truth, and hope. I have been lucky enough to say blessings many times.

Personally, I like to combine ideas from many faiths. There is
the Jewish concept of how food sustains us to reach another day.
There is the Buddhist ideal of asking that all beings are free from
hunger. There is the Islamic ideal of taking care that no neighbors
go hungry. Then, there is the Christian philosophy on using the
energy that food gives us to bring service to others. And, there is the
Hindu idea of hospitality and giving thanks for bringing people
together.

Ritual blessings are appetizers for your mindful meal. Just as
appetizers change, you need not have the same blessing each time.

◆

What mealtime blessing idea is most
important for you to express at today's meal?

Eating

The full use of taste is an act of genius.

JOHN LA FARGE, ARTIST

THE FULL USE OF TASTE IS NOT ONLY GENIUS. It is miraculous. The enzyme amylase, which is present in saliva, begins to digest carbohydrates as you grind and chew your food. Chewing also breaks food into smaller pieces that come into contact with the taste buds.

How many times do you chew? There is no right answer. In mindfulness training, Buddhist monks practice chewing food from twenty-five to a hundred times prior to swallowing. The more attention you place on chewing, the more you will taste your food with greater intensity and bliss.

This practice is best done in silence. Begin with something small, like a raisin, a grape, an almond, or a slice of orange. Take small bites. Be mindful as you chew, feeling how the food taste and consistency keep changing.

I have had people tell me that a raisin, for example, tasted different at the end than in the middle. Expect the unexpected.

◆

Chew a snack mindfully twenty-five
times before swallowing.

Community

*Forgiveness is to offer no resistance to life – to
allow life to live through you. The alternatives are
pain and suffering.*

ECKHART TOLLE, *The Power of Now*

WHAT DOES IT MEAN TO FORGIVE AT MEALTIME?
If you hold a grudge during a meal, it will affect how you eat.
If you are tense, then you may eat more quickly and chew less,
which will affect your digestion. If you are upset with someone
during mealtime – whether or not they are present – you may stop
listening to your body's signals and eat more (or less) food than
you need.

Forgiving, like eating, is a healing and nourishing experience. If
you hold a grudge or anger toward another, then you are only continuing your suffering. What are you holding onto?

Mealtime is a good time to learn to forgive and let go. The food
on your table gives itself to you voluntarily. You ritual blessing for-
gives you for your own mistakes. After all, who has not erred in life?

◆

Let go of anger, even a little. Forgive as you
are forgiven at the dinner table.

Departure

*The more one lets go, the stronger the presence
of the Spirit becomes. The Ultimate Mystery
becomes the Ultimate Presence.*

FATHER THOMAS KEATING, *Open Mind, Open Heart*

LETTING GO OF MEALTIME EMOTIONS CAN SOME-
times require forgiveness for oneself. How do you forgive
yourself for mindlessly eating, for example?

After all, who is to blame for your eating issues? Do you blame
your parents, your caregivers, and others for saddling you with eating problems? Yes, you may be absolutely correct that they had a
role in it – but now, as an adult, you need to do something for yourself. You might want the person who did this to you to suffer, but
will that help your eating issue?

Forgiving does not mean forgetting. But it does mean that you
are ready to let go, to move beyond your hurt and your pain and
to start living in the present again. This is something you need to
do for your own well-being.

◆

How do forgiveness of food
issues set you free?

Entry

A sensation of hunger is the body's built-in clock, telling you it's time to eat.

DEBORAH KESTEN,
Feeding the Body, Nourishing the Soul

YOUR BODY OPERATES IN TUNE WITH WHAT IS called a circadian rhythm, or a twenty-four-hour biological cycle. These rhythms affect your sleep, hormones, and hunger. Other things can affect hunger, like changes in the body's blood glucose level.

You might not be able to know when your hormones and glucose level go up or down and cause hunger, but you can feel those times when hunger is cued by your environment, stress, and other causes that have nothing to do with biological hunger.

If you go straight for the refrigerator or make unscheduled stops at the convenience store after a stress-filled day, you need to engage your awareness. Get in the habit of taking short breaks to breathe into your diaphragm for three minutes – to reduce your stress level. Then, make sure you have a healthy snack in your car at all times.

◆

Recognize the difference between biological and stress hunger. Lower stress with mindful breathing and healthy snacks.

Choices

The path of freedom
Does not lead to the goal of freedom;
It is the path of discipline
Which leads to the goal of liberty.

INAYAT KHAN, *Notes from the Unstuck Music*

To HAVE FREEDOM IN YOUR FOOD CHOICES MEANS that you discern and choose wisely those foods that give you longevity and health. Freedom does not mean eating everything and anything regardless of the consequences. There needs to be some boundaries on your eating, at least as you begin to gain the strength to make wise choices.

On the day that balanced, blissful eating comes naturally, you will eat what you want, and as much as you know to be nonharmful. Until then, use discipline to build up your strength.

Do not make the mistake of thinking that discipline is an all-or-none proposition. You cannot suddenly hope to cut out a food habit with years of power behind it. Make changes slowly. Be kind to yourself! Enact little changes that you succeed at.

◆

What is the smallest change in my eating
that can I make today and succeed at?

Preparations

No failure is ever really a failure unless we stop
trying altogether – indeed, it may be a blessing in
disguise, a much-needed lesson.

SWAMI PRABHAVANANDA AND CHRISTOPHER
ISHERWOOD, *How to Know God*

 DID YOU EVER MAKE A MEAL THAT WAS, TO PUT it gently, a flop? These humbling experiences prove one thing. You are human. A perfect omelet is not mastered in a day. From my brief experience rolling sushi, for example, it took weeks of practice until I learned how to cover the nori (seaweed) with just the right amount of rice and put enough crab, cucumber, and avocado inside so that it would close nicely.

Perhaps it does not matter if you ever get it right. What is important is that you learn to be tolerant with yourself and accepting of mistakes. This also means tolerance toward others – your partner, friend, child, or roommate – who might help you prepare a meal.

Let yourself "ripen" as you prepare, learning more about yourself in the process.

✦

What one new thing can you learn about
preparation and cooking today?

Rituals

God will not change the condition of a people
Until they change what is in their hearts.

QU'RAN 13:11

 WHAT DOES YOUR HEART TELL YOU DURING your mealtime ritual? Are you frightened by food? Resentful at having to eat with another? Angry for cheating on your well-crafted eating plan? Shamed because you do not like your body weight or size?

So long as you do not acknowledge these feelings at your ritual blessing, it will be difficult to move past them. Healing begins with acknowledgment.

Begin by stating and experiencing your honest feelings before you eat. You might even want to add something like this to your ritual blessing: "Though this meal is not calorie-free, may this meal be free of guilt and shame. I can always be guilty another time if I choose. But now I choose to eat in peace."

◆

Choose to eat a meal in peace by
acknowledging and letting your feelings be.

Eating

Why put off till tomorrow what you can eat today?
MISS PIGGY, MUPPET PUPPET CHARACTER

JUST WHEN YOU THINK IT IS SAFE TO GO IN THE kitchen you find yourself feeling like Miss Piggy. Fortunately, you can substitute quality for quantity by satisfying yourself with mindfulness of sensation.

Five minutes before your meal, get a grape, baby carrot, celery stick, or other small fruit or vegetable. Examine it closely. Think how it grew out of the ground. What did the young plant look like? How long did it take to mature and ripen? Look closely at its color, shape, size, and texture. Does it have an aroma?

Take a tiny bite. Is it crunchy or soft? Can you taste or feel any "skin" on it? Is it sweet? Tart? What feelings and thoughts arise as you chew? Appreciate how this food is absorbed and digested by your body. Continue this for up to five minutes, appreciating, savoring, and exploring each little bite. Now, extend this mindfulness to your meal.

◆

Five minutes before your meal,
savor a food mindfully.

Community

You must remember, and teach your children, that
the rivers are our brothers, and yours, and you
must henceforth give the rivers the kindness you
would give to any brother.

PARAPHRASE OF CHIEF SEATTLE

DO YOU RECYCLE YOUR PLASTIC, GLASS, AND CANS after a meal? Do you make an effort to use cleaning products and dishwashing detergents that are easy on the environment?

By your actions you set a powerful example. When you are careful about not wasting resources, for example, you teach conservation. By not wasting food you make a statement that it is valuable. If it is important enough to give you life, then it is important enough to conserve and use wisely.

Even when disposing of food, think about what you can do with it. Donate your unused canned goods to food banks. Let neighbors know you care by giving a gift of food the next time you visit.

◆

Waste not; want not. How can you more
consciously conserve food?

Departure

To eat is human; to digest, divine.

CHARLES T. COPELAND

HAVE YOU NOTICED THAT THE ONLY TIME YOU think about your digestion is when it is not working optimally? It does not seem fair that eating gets all the glory while digestion does all the work.

What foods are difficult for you to digest? Being mindful of this might even bring up a difficult memory around such an occurence. Should this happen, you may recognize a pattern of how well you digest different foods.

If you cannot process the foods on a particular diet, then that diet may not be best for you. Likewise, if you have digestion problems, talk to a nutritionist or registered dietician about how a new diet might improve your digestion. Fortunately, there are many acceptable substitutes for most foods.

◆

Let your digestion guide the direction
of your food intake.

Entry

No man is lonely while eating spaghetti –
it requires too much attention

CHRISTOPHER MORLEY,
U.S. AUTHOR AND JOURNALIST

How do you feel about eating alone? Do you prefer company or do you enjoy dining solo? The truth is that no one needs to be lonely or alone while eating. As you prepare for your meal, bring present-moment awareness and other tools with you to your breakfast, lunch, dinner, or snack.

The divine is always present through the miracle of food and your awareness. You can accentuate this by placing your attention on all the beneficial aspects of your upcoming meal.

For example, how can your surroundings enhance your experience? Even if you eat in an office cubicle, you can arrange the space to make it more than a work area. Create a sacred dining space by putting up a picture of trees, a river, a mountain, or other inspiring photo. Take a moment of silence to appreciate the meal and the space you are entering.

◆

Enter sacred dining by making
your space sacred.

Choices

Routine in cuisine is crime.

ÉDOUARD NIGNON, AUTHOR

 DO YOU ALWAYS HAVE A CUP OF COFFEE, A MUFFIN, or a bagel and cream cheese for breakfast? Daily food routines are convenient, save time, and offer predictable safety. On the other hand, they can also slide into mindless eating and the possibility of addictive behavior. If how you eat feels frozen or causes you health problems, then you may want to seriously consider changing your routine.

You do not have to jettison all of your eating routine at once. For example, coffee was part of my morning routine. But the more I drank, the more I felt myself losing energy. Eventually, I realized that coffee gave me a short-term boost but a long-term energy deficit. I altered my routine by substituting tea and decaf, only drinking an occasional cup of "real" coffee, and now I feel much better.

◆

Be bold and vary your eating routine away
from mindless and addictive behavior.

Preparations

Idleness is the enemy of the soul.

SAINT BENEDICT, *The Rule of St. Benedict*

 HOW DO YOU FEEL ABOUT KITCHEN AND MEAL preparation work? Do you dislike manual labor of any kind? Do you feel that cleaning or preparing food is a job better left to others? If so, then you may miss tapping in to the sacred that exists in plain sight in your kitchen.

In our culture, we are often led to believe that work around cooking and cleaning is best to be avoided. So many "labor-saving" devices are supposed to take the drudgery out of mealtime. The message here is that certain kitchen tasks are meaningless and you cannot find anything of value in them. How far from the truth this is.

Being fully present with any task can transform it from the mundane to the sublime. Watch your attitudes. Do not let preconceived ideas steal away meaningful labor.

◆

Transform your attitudes about kitchen work.

Rituals

I vow to understand living beings and their
suffering, to cultivate compassion and loving
kindness, and to practice joy and equanimity.

THICH NHAT HANH

ARE YOU SO BUSY THROUGHOUT THE DAY THAT you rarely have time to go "deep" with your feelings and understanding of others? Mealtime is the perfect time to extend your thoughts to others via reflection, prayer, and ritual blessing.

When you "vow to understand living beings and their suffering," you enter a place of communication and communion. You step outside yourself and recognize the connection between yourself and others. In Buddhism, there is the idea that when "one hummingbird is fed, all beings are fed." Likewise, when one child starves, all beings starve.

During your ritual blessing, take the reality of starvation and suffering close to heart. This will open your heart, not harden it. Rest in loving kindness, compassion, joy, and equanimity – even for a moment – and your meal will be sublime.

◆

Use your mealtime moment to understand
others and cultivate compassion and joy.

Eating

*Not long ago, there was a fad in certain New York
restaurants for the guaranteed thirty-minute
lunch.... If that isn't a recipe for tension and
indigestion, I'll swallow my cell phone.*

PETER MAYLE, *Encore Provence*

I DO NOT KNOW ABOUT YOU, BUT I HAVE SEEN A few people practically swallow their cell phones during lunch. Eating quickly and talking on the cell phone, however, do not bring balance to food and eating.

In their book *The Power of Full Engagement*, authors Jim Loehr and Tony Schwartz describe how the body undergoes a natural cycle every ninety minutes. During this time, the blood pressure and blood sugar levels drop. They conclude that you need rest periods throughout the day, especially while eating.

Do not give in to the temptation to keep running nonstop. The only one who may suffer is you – from exhaustion, fatigue, and irritability. Try planning several healthy snacks throughout the day. This could break an existing cycle of eating and give your body the support it needs.

◆

Slow yourself down at today's meal.
Simply eat and eat simply.

Community

*My wife and I tried to breakfast together,
but we had to stop or our marriage would
have been wrecked.*

WINSTON CHURCHILL

WHAT IS YOUR STYLE OF EATING WITH OTHERS? Are you the silent and grumpy type? Or, perhaps you are wound up with energy, full of optimism, and ready to talk up a storm. Incompatible eating styles are just that: incompatible. It is unlikely that another person will change to suit your mealtime needs and temperament.

If there is someone in your life that you do not mix well with at mealtime, here is a suggestion. Call a truce. Even if the other person is unaware of this, you can still call a truce by suspending your own annoyance during the meal. Discover the limits of your patience and forbearance, and then try to extend these a step further.

And, if you are mindful of your emotional cycles, you might choose to have breakfast alone, but have other meals in the company of others.

✦

Be in tune with your emotional cycles and
have a peaceful meal alone or with others.

Departure

I know people who'd rather throw out food than
eat leftovers the next day. Poor deprived souls.

SHARON TYLER HERBST, AUTHOR

 FOR SOME, LEFTOVERS ARE ASSOCIATED WITH poverty. For others, they signify a treasure that is not to be wasted. It seems that people either love leftovers or hate them.

After a meal, what do you do with your leftovers? Do you consistently eat more than you want to avoid leftovers and feel guilty about it? Do you cringe at the idea of reheated food? Or do you find ways of combining your leftovers to make a new and unique meal? In this sense, leftovers may tell you more about yourself and your willingness to adapt.

Even if you cannot stand to eat leftovers, you can still find a way to offer the food to others. A gift of food to another is almost always appreciated with love and joy.

◆

Give leftovers to a neighbor or other person.

Entry

In the Middle Ages, they had guillotines,
stretch racks, whips and chains. Nowadays, we
have a much more effective torture device called
the bathroom scale.

STEPHEN PHILLIPS, WRITER

WHEN YOU ENTER THE MEALTIME SPACE, DO you worry about weight and diet? Do you count the calories and think about weighing yourself after your meal? If so, then you have instituted a torture device of your own making.

What is behind these thoughts? Pay attention to your mind. Do you have internal scripts that play out worries and anxieties and insecurities?

Some scripts, for example, might sound like this:"If I do not look good, then no one will love me.""I am not really lovable or attractive.""I feel empty inside and I need a way to feel good and fill myself up."

Adopt a new positive script as you enter your meal:"I am a human being who deserves love.""I am worthwhile and precious." "I do not need food to comfort me because I am already complete and whole."

◆

At today's meal, be aware of your
old script. Practice a new positive one
or create your own.

Choices

It has always seemed strange to me that
people can be vague and casual about what
they put into their mouths.

PAMELA VANDYKE PRICE, WRITER

WHEN YOU THINK ABOUT IT, THERE ARE FEW things as intimate as eating. It is intimate because there are limited ways for substances to enter the body. So when you are talking about food, you are really getting personal!

Choosing food can be just as personal, since your choice will be ingested in short order. So how can you do this as lovingly as possible? How can you select your own food with love and care?

Here is one way: As the seasons shift you can be more mindful of the foods your body craves as it adapts to climatic changes. Find balance and harmony between your body and nature by preparing ingredients that you know to be pure and fresh and seasonal. Some good spring foods, for example, include wild mushrooms, corn, cherry tomatoes, and strawberries. If you are unsure, ask your local produce manager what foods are seasonal.

◆

Reflect on the intimacy of food and how this
influences your preparation.

Preparations

Go into the kitchen to shake the chef's hand.
If he is thin, have second thoughts about eating
there; if he is thin and sad, flee.

FERNAND POINT, CHEF

PERSONALLY, I WOULD NOT WORRY SO MUCH ABOUT whether the chef at your favorite restaurant is generously proportioned or thin. I might, however, have second thoughts if the chef is perpetually frowning, miserable, annoyed, angry, and pessimistic.

Think about yourself for a moment. How do you prepare food when you are in a bad mood, anxious, or depressed? Since your mood affects how you touch, feel, listen, and experience the world, your emotional energy may also mix with the food you prepare.

Think about the last time you were in a great mood or a bad one. Can you remember a meal you ate during each occasion? Perhaps an upset mood altered the delicate flavors of your food? Or, maybe you lost your appetite altogether. If so, it is not really surprising.

Be the chef who brings optimism and hope into the kitchen and into your meal.

◆

Cook today's meal with a smile.

Rituals

*I pray that we may at all times keep our
minds open to new ideas and shun dogma; that we
may grow in our understanding of the nature
of all living beings and our connectedness with
the natural world.*

JANE GOODALL, WILDLIFE BIOLOGIST

 YOU CAN TAILOR ALMOST ANY RITUAL BLESSING
or prayer to support and encourage a specific aspect of how
you eat. Jane Goodall's blessing, for example, can help you open
your mind to new eating ideas.

Have you ignored an important food source because you are
stuck being only a pasta lover, a bread lover, or a meat lover? A ritual blessing that helps you set the intention for eating another kind
of food could be useful and beneficial.

Did you know, for instance, that the National Cancer Institute
recommends five servings of fruit and vegetables daily? You could
add a phrase such as "May I be blessed with enough fruits and vegetables for my mind and body" to your present blessing.

This will also gently remind you to have more fruit and vegetables throughout the day.

+

What beneficial foods can your ritual
blessing give you permission to eat?

Eating

Even a single day of a life lived virtuously and
meditatively is worth more than a hundred years
lived wantonly and without discipline.

THE BUDDHA, *Dhammapada*

TAKING THE BUDDHA'S CUE, A SINGLE MEAL eaten meditatively is worth more than a hundred meals eaten without discipline or mindfulness. For today's meditation, you will get the chance to use discipline by pausing before eating.

Do you ever go to a Mexican restaurant and fill up on chips before the meal arrives? (Who hasn't?) And the reason is simple: Your entire focus, concentration, and hunger are directed at the only food source on the table – those poor chips that you want to devour. Fortunately, you can overcome this obstacle at any meal – and not by denying yourself the chips.

Here's how: Give yourself permission to eat all the chips you want! The catch is this: You must wait until after the entrée arrives at the table. Once your food is served, the chips are rarely as appealing. You aren't denying yourself anything. You are just pausing with discipline.

◆

Wait until more foods are on
the table before eating.

Community

As we share in the breaking of bread . . . as we share words, I am also breaking my life, I am breaking open my memory and sharing it with others, and they with me.

JEAN MOLESKY-POZ, FORMER FRANCISCAN MONK

EATING WITH ANOTHER IS A FORM OF INTIMACY. Because of this, eating with others also raises some worry and anxiety. What if I order the wrong thing? What if I eat too much or too little? What if my dinner conversation is trite or boring?

There are many what-ifs that can present themselves at community meals. But with mindfulness you can always set the intention to be yourself. You can set the intention to share some of your life and memory without judgment as you break bread with another. Then, just enjoy the meal.

In any event, you need to accept this: You cannot predict what another will think of how you eat. Know that everyone is criticized or judged. There was an occasion, for example, when the Buddha's monks disagreed with him and walked out on him! So you are in good company.

And if you do not want to talk, you can always listen, which is a gift you can offer another.

◆

Be aware of what-ifs when dining today. Then set the intention to be present with your meal.

Departure

Ego is not sin.
Ego is not something that you get rid of.
Ego is something that you come to know.

PEMA CHÖDRÖN, *Start Where You Are*

HAVE YOU EVER MENTALLY AND EMOTIONALLY beaten yourself up after a meal? Chances are that your statements fall into one of several ego-blaming categories.

First is guilt: "I shouldn't have eaten that extra helping." Next is seeing your eating patterns as all or nothing: "I'll never have control over my eating," or "I'll always be overweight." Then there is emotional overload, which could sound like: "I'm so upset that I can't stay on a healthy eating plan anyway."

Is it really true, for example, that you never have control over your eating or never make a healthy food choice? Get to know yourself better not by blaming, but by broadening your limited narrow thoughts about how you eat. There is always another side to every picture.

◆

Be mindful of blame around food.

Entry

Nothing helps scenery like ham and eggs.

MARK TWAIN

ENTERING THE DAY WITHOUT FOOD IS LIKE running your car on empty. Sooner or later, you will be forced to stop and fill up. But do you really want to wait for an emergency appetite before eating?

Many years ago, breakfast was an important staple of the American diet. Today, life is fast-paced, and more people in the household may be working. The result, all too often, is a missed breakfast.

As Mark Twain suggested, however, a breakfast may help your "scenery" at work or school by making you more productive, alert, and centered. If you do not currently eat breakfast, change this routine for just one day by having a complete breakfast consisting of a broad choice of foods. Note the changes and see if this gives you a smoother transition into your daily activities.

◆

Take time for a breakfast.

Choices

Skillful farmers do better than random farmers.

LAMA SURYA DAS

WHAT FOODS WOULD BE IN YOUR SHOPPING cart if you randomly selected items off the shelf? You might end up with all bread, all fruit, or all canned corn. A skillful farmer does not plant seeds in winter or harvest in spring. Likewise, you need to be skillful when it comes to choosing your meals and crafting a balanced diet.

As women age, for example, there is loss of bone density. Some studies have shown that vitamin K may decrease hip fractures in older women. So you may want to include more dark green vegetables, like broccoli and spinach – which are rich in vitamin K – into your diet.

By skillfully planning your diet, you plant the seeds of vibrant health and well-being. This also encourages you to explore the idea of prevention in terms of heading off potential problems.

◆

Skillfully choose the foods
that bring you health.

Preparations

*Food imaginatively and lovingly prepared, and
eaten in good company, warms the being with
something more than the mere intake of calories.*

MARJORIE KINNAN RAWLINGS

 FOOD PREPARATION SOMETIMES MEANS WORKING
with others. Have you ever prepared a meal with another?
If you share cooking and preparation duties, how you coordinate
tasks and responsibilities can make all the difference between harmony and acrimony.

There is some truth in the well-worn phrase, "too many cooks
spoil the broth." What this really means is that narrow-mindedness
and noncooperation ruin the ability to create and prepare anything
– especially a meal.

Are you possessive about the way you create food? Do you have
to be in charge? Become aware of these tendencies. When you invite someone into your kitchen preparation – or if you are invited –
become mindful of using kind words, open communication, and
a spirit of sharing. You can take this approach even if you are cooking for others who instruct you how to make their food.

◆

Create harmony in meal preparation
with others by cooperating and being
less in charge.

Rituals

*Let us invoke our ancestors, both spiritual
and genetic. For we are the sole reason
for their existence.*

ROSHI JOHN DAIDO LOORI, ZEN TEACHER

THE ABOVE MEALTIME RITUAL BLESSING – OR ONE like it – is ideal for acknowledging and giving thanks to those who came before. In particular, do you have a grandparent or great grandparent who made a difference in your life who you would like to remember and thank? Maybe you have a relative who showed you kindness around food.

Personally, I am still touched by the actions of my Grandmother Martha, who lovingly made me lunch almost each day one summer when I lived near her retirement apartment in Florida. She insisted I come, and she always baked something special, like pecan cookies or bread.

Take a moment to thank those who fed and nourished you as you grew up. This addition to the mealtime ritual connects you to your past and to all the positive aspects of food through which love is given.

✦

Add a ritual blessing of thanks to an
ancestor, relative, or other person.

Eating

It is wonderful, if we chose the right diet, what an extraordinarily small quantity would suffice.

GANDHI

DO YOU ALWAYS ORDER OR PREPARE A BIG MEAL for lunch or dinner? In the United States, where meals seem to be getting bigger, it may be helpful to ask how much food you really need.

Have you ever dieted or restricted your food intake, even for a short period of time? If so, then you probably know, as did Gandhi – who learned how to fast from his mother and undertook several prolonged fasts – that you can live on a lot less food than you ever imagined.

At a convenience mart or restaurant, you might get more food than you want. Do you eat the entire meal because it gives you an excuse to do so? Or because you do not like to waste food?

Eat what you need by taking food home or sharing one meal with a friend.

◆

Consciously eat a little less food
at today's meal.

Community

There's more. Eat up. Eat all you want. There's all
the rolls in the world here.

RAYMOND CARVER, *A Small Good Thing*

HAVE YOU EVER GIVEN FOOD TO A FAMILY OR person who was grieving or suffering? If so, then you have taken part in an ancient community tradition. Food is often used as a means of support during times of hardship and grief.

In the Chinese tradition, for example, there is a "day of remembrance" to honor and remember ancestors. On this day, families traditionally offer food and share a meal together.

In the Jewish tradition, friends and families bring baskets of food to those who have lost a loved one. It is known as a "meal of recovery." Hindus, Muslims, and others have similar customs.

Even if you do not follow or adhere to any specific tradition, you can adapt the practice to add richness to your life.

✦

Be aware of how you can support those who
suffer or grieve with the gift of food.

Departure

*Live in simple faith . . . just as this trusting
cherry flowers, fades, and falls.*

ISSA, POET

HAVE YOU EVER SAID THANK YOU TO FRIENDS
for inviting you to their home for dinner? You can think of
it as a kind of departure blessing. This is a good way to transition
from mealtime into what comes next.

In some cultures and traditions this departure is formalized.
The Sabbath, for example, is sometimes concluded with the sweet
smell of nutmeg and other spices – which represents hope for the
week ahead.

How can you depart your meal with a sense of optimism, hope,
and faith? First, pause for a moment to appreciate the meal you have
just finished. Realize that food has provided for your spiritual,
mental, and physical needs and dreams.

You are the beautiful flower that has just been watered and
nourished by your meal.

◆

Leave your meal with gratitude
and appreciation.

Entry

*Right now today, could you make an
unconditional relationship with yourself? Just at
the height you are, the weight you are, the
amount of intelligence that you have, the burden
of pain that you have?*

PEMA CHÖDRÖN, *Start Where Your Are*

WHAT IS IN YOUR THOUGHTS AS YOU ENTER mealtime? Is your mind filled up with conditions for loving yourself? Do you withhold your love – waiting for the moment when you are the right height, weight, or body shape? If so, think of the love you are missing right now.

What would it take for you to drop the conditions, even a little? What would help you become more unconditional with yourself – even if you are having a "bad meal day"?

Know this: No matter how much you may feel unloved in your life, you are worthy of an unconditional relationship.

Your conditional thoughts have been acquired over time. You can let yourself hear them and feel them without judgment. Know, too, that the conditional thought is not the same as you. Unconditionally, you can simply accept yourself as you are.

◆

Observe your conditional thoughts. Accept
yourself in unconditional relationship.

Choices

*You can pour Ajax in the tub and leave it there
for days or weeks, but unless you scrub with some
real elbow power, nothing gets cleaned.*

DONALD ALTMAN, *Living Kindness*

ARE YOU LAZY WITH YOUR FOOD CHOICES? Do you accept less than what you deserve? Do you take the easy road, the metaphorical fast-food lane, because you do not have to think about it?

Imagine for a moment that you are stressed out and hungry. Now, without giving it too much thought, think of the first food choice or restaurant that comes to mind. Whatever your answer, know that you do not have to have that same knee-jerk reaction in real life.

At this moment, I want you to again imagine feeling stressed and hungry. As before, picture the first food or restaurant that pops into your head. Now, however, take a long, mindful breath and set the intention: May I choose foods that will nourish me fully at this moment. Allow yourself to substitute a different food or restaurant in your mind's eye. Visualize yourself eating this new choice.

◆

Make an intentional food
or meal choice today.

Preparations

*One of the first requisites of a tea master is
knowledge of how to sweep, clean, and wash, for
there is an art in cleaning and dusting.*

KAKUZO OKAKURA, *The Book of Tea*

HAVE YOU EVER GONE ABOUT PREPARING YOUR meal mechanically, on autopilot? When this happens, you may not really see the beauty of what is in your own kitchen and surroundings that can enhance your meal preparation.

This reminds me of the story of boy who was told to clean the path in front of his parent's small restaurant. He swept and swept, removing every little twig and leaf until the walk was immaculate and free of debris. And yet, his father was not happy with the results. When the boy asked why, his father said, "True cleaning always leaves some innate, natural beauty."

A Japanese tea room, for example, is constructed of natural wood and decorated with a *chabana*, or elegant flower arrangement, with colors to signify a theme.

◆

What touch of nature can you add
to your meal preparation?

Rituals

Pray for peace and grace and spiritual food,
For wisdom and guidance, for all these are good.
But don't forget the potatoes.

JOHN TYLER PETEE, *Prayer and Potatoes*

HOW DOES YOUR RITUAL MEALTIME BLESSING touch you? Does it transport you into a sacred realm? Or does it keep you grounded in the reality of food and eating? Both aspects are equally important, and both show how mealtime ritual brings the sacred and mundane harmoniously together.

In addition to inviting the sacred, a mealtime prayer can give you new insight into your meal. Here is how: As you prepare to intone your ritual blessing, place your attention on the food at the table. Take a moment to scan the choices that are available. You can also do this after the blessing, giving you a moment to experience what foods speak to you.

Let your body tune in to these foods and resonate with them. Then, fully appreciate the web of being that connects you, the earth, and the food that sustains you. Select foods that your intuition tells you are best for you at this moment.

◆

Experience the sacred and mundane
of food with your blessing.

Eating

Seeing is deceiving. It's eating that's believing.

JAMES THURBER, *Further Fables for Our Times*

SEEING ONLY ENGAGES ONE OF YOUR SENSES. BUT food is a powerful sensual experience that engages all your senses. No wonder you are seduced by the sight, smell, taste, and touch of it. (Also, you can hear the sound of food as you chew it.)

For this meditation, practice being mindful of all your senses. (1) Use your sight to look at food's color and shape with full concentration. (2) Smell a food's aroma – both cooked and uncooked. Can you tell when something is fresh or spoiled? (3) Taste a food by letting it linger in your mouth for a long time, chewing it and extracting all the flavor it has to give you. Do you like or dislike it? (4) Experience details of a food's texture and sound as you chew. (5) Hear food as you crunch, munch, and pop it in your mouth.

+

Experience food deeply, with all your senses.

Community

He asked Jesus, "And who is my neighbor?"

LUKE 10:29

WHEN IT COMES TO FOOD AND EATING, WHO IS
your true neighbor? The Bible story of the Good Samaritan
answers this way: It is one who is willing to offer food to someone –
even a stranger – who is distressed or suffering. In real life, though,
showing kindness to a stranger through food can be frightening.

I know a well-to-do family that enjoys every major convenience.
Each year during Thanksgiving, however, the parents take their
children to a homeless shelter where the whole family participates
in feeding the homeless. One of the parents said, "I want our kids
to know that there are people who have less and who need help."

Can you show mercy and find your comfort zone at the same
time? Maybe you cannot. Still, you can face your fears and share
food with your less fortunate neighbors when the opportunity
arises.

✦

You do not have to change the world. You
can simply open your eyes and become less
judgmental of those in need.

Departure

If you let go a little, you will have a little happiness.
If you let go a lot, you will have a lot of happiness.
If you let go completely, you will be free.

ACHAAN CHAH, BUDDHIST MONK

WHEN YOU DEPART FROM MEALTIME, DO YOU STILL think about food? If you are on a diet regimen, for example, you may still be hungry or feeling unsatisfied. Or perhaps you are thinking about how to do a better job of sticking to your dietary needs at the next meal.

When this is the case, my suggestion is as follows: Instead of living in the past, consciously embrace this now moment of noneating. Sometimes it is easier to let go of something if you replace it with a substitute. Since your eating is done, you can naturally embrace noneating between meals.

Think of your space between meals as a periodic, or temporary, fast, which has many benefits. As used in many traditions, periodic fasting gives your entire body a rest. A vow to keep your periodic fast until the next meal strengthens concentration and limits snacking.

✦

Embrace noneating between meals.

Entry

For if you bake bread with indifference, you bake
a bitter bread that feeds but half our hunger.

KAHLIL GIBRAN, *The Prophet*

DO YOU EVER APPROACH MEALTIME AS IF IT were an annoyance, something to get out of the way so you could move on to more important things? Do you come to a meal with an attitude of indifference or ambivalence because you just want to get it over with?

This approach might save a few extra minutes, but it might also keep you from satisfying your hunger, because eating represents a metaphor for feeding yourself at all levels – from the emotional to the financial.

If you routinely feel indifferent about your upcoming meal, then this may indicate a lack of self-love or self-nurturing that needs to be healed. Become aware of when you feel like this. When did you first develop this attitude? What would it feel like to appreciate your meals?

◆

Reflect on mealtime indifference and what
meal appreciation feels like.

Choices

Mammals are "supersmellers,"
with the best noses in the business.

LYALL WATSON,
Jacobson's Organ and the Remarkable Nature of Smell

RECENTLY, MY WIFE AND I VISITED AN OUTDOOR mall that contained several restaurants. We stepped into several to check out the menus. But we were still undecided until we entered a restaurant filled with the most delicious aroma. "Let's eat here," I said instantly.

Have you ever had a sensual experience like this one? If you are ever unsure about what food to choose, let your highly developed sense of smell help you decide. It can, for example, help you determine if products such as dairy, fish, and meat are spoiled or fresh. It can also help you tell if some fruits or vegetables are ripened to perfection.

Be more mindful and attuned to using your nose. It can help you tap into what foods your energy body might require at this instant.

◆

Use your sense of smell to help you choose
foods for today's meal.

Preparations

Create a visual feast as well as an edible one.

DARLENE JONES, *Cooking with Spirit*

THINK BACK TO A SPECIAL MEAL IN YOUR LIFE – either at a restaurant or in someone's home. Do you recall the ambiance? Did it give you a feeling of warmth and joy that enhanced the meal?

Holiday, anniversary, and birthday meals are notable not just for the food. A birthday celebration, for example, is also made special because of the thoughtfully placed decorations, the decorated cake, and festive table settings.

You do not need a special occasion to make your table setting and ambiance sacred and meaningful. The warmth and appeal of your home serve as a mindful appetizer for any meal that focuses you on the moment. Toward that end, think about using scented candles or aroma therapy to prepare and enhance the setting. Herbs, flowers, and other plants can also make your dining space inviting.

✦

Add something new to your
mealtime ambiance.

Rituals

Improve yourself for your own sake,
and people will follow you.

ARISTOTLE

DO YOU RECITE A RITUAL MEALTIME BLESSING because you have always done so? Do you feel it is an obligation? Or do you do so because it is important to you?

At my own home or in restaurants, for example, I often like to create a unique mealtime blessing to fit the moment. Maybe there is someone new who is sharing this meal, or perhaps the meal itself commemorates a special occasion. The point here is that you can bring the now moment into your mealtime blessing at each meal.

In this way, you promote a mindful attitude, rather than just reciting a blessing by rote memory. Anything done by rote – whether eating or reciting a blessing – tends to remove you from the mindful moment. When your blessing connects to the moment it becomes alive and fresh.

Who knows? You might even inspire others to do the same with their blessings.

◆

Explore why you say a blessing. At today's
meal, do it for yourself.

Eating

*If you want a quick way to see how people relate
to God, watch the way they eat.*

BROTHER ALAN, O.H.C.

WHEN BROTHER ALAN, A JOVIAL, GRAY-HAIRED monk, said this to me, I had to laugh! I could immediately see what he meant. Since food is an expression and creation of the divine, how can your relationship to food and the divine be separate things?

While watching others is fascinating, it is also useful to watch yourself. If your style of eating reflected how you relate to the divine, what would that relationship be? How would you want to change it?

Use mindfulness to create the relationship you want – with food and the divine. Set an intention before each bite. Follow up with action. Then, observe your thoughts and senses while eating. Let nothing escape your net of awareness. Be deeply present and grateful as you ingest the divine energy of food with each bite.

◆

Watch your own relationship with food
and eating through mindfulness.

Community

*Never argue at the dinner table, for the one who is
not hungry always gets the best of the argument.*
RICHARD WHATLEY

 HAVE YOU EVER ARGUED OVER A MEAL? OR SAID
something you regretted? If so, you know firsthand that a
mealtime argument causes both the "winner" and "loser" to lose.

Mealtime is an excellent time to practice patience and openness – both with eating and with others. Patience cannot really be
experienced without the virtues of forgiveness, forbearance, and
kindness.

If you cannot be patient, then you can explore the roots of your
impatience. Sometimes, personal hurt, anger, and expectation can
cause impatience. Observing the unkind dinner remarks of others
(or yourself) is a good first step. Then, do what you can to forgive
(or ask for forgiveness) in the moment. If you cannot do that, then
search deeper for the reasons you were unkind or impatient.

◆

Practice patience, forbearance,
and kindness at today's meal.

Departure

Better to light a candle than to curse the darkness.

CONFUCIUS

YOU MIGHT WANT TO THINK OF YOUR EMOTIONS and struggles that you hold onto after your meal as "darkness." But the moment you recognize the truth of how they judge you and others, you have a "candle" that brings light into your life.

You do not need to depart your meal with emotional angst, frustration, and conflict over what you did or did not eat. You do not need to carry the calorie count with you as a reminder of how you failed. Rather, accept these thoughts for what they are: one limited view of things at this moment.

Besides, your thoughts are not really permanent, but temporary. Observe closely and you will find that each thought has a beginning, middle, and end. Like the clouds in the sky, just watch them come and go without clinging to them. Let this be your illuminating candle for today.

◆

Light a candle of awareness to your
emotions after today's meal.

Entry

*Take time to declare a happy hunting
ground in your house and in your feelings,
and hunt there everyday.*

Don Gerrard, *One Bowl*

Do you ever look in your cupboards and find something you had forgotten about which delights you? Consider your kitchen or a restaurant a "happy hunting ground" in which to find new treasures. The secret to making this happen is in your attitude.

Think back to a time that you anticipated going to a meal. Were you visiting a new restaurant that got a wonderful review? Were you about to eat one of your favorite foods? Were you going to meet someone you had not seen in a long, long time? Know that you can recreate that feeling of excitement around your next meal.

Begin by setting the intention to have a special meal. This could be anything from cooking or preparing something different to inviting a new friend to dinner. However large or small the change, do something that brings you joy and makes you smile.

♦

Set the intention to bring joy into your meal.

Choices

Food is wisdom for the soul.

DONALD ALTMAN

WHAT IS THE MOST EXOTIC AND UNUSUAL FOOD you have ever tasted? Do you know, for example, that even the "common" apple consists of 2,000 different varieties? From sweet to tart and in all colors, apples are just one example of food's wonderful diversity. Have you explored Fuji, Swiss Gourmet, Golden Russet, and Gold, just to name a few? In fact, the ancient Greeks domesticated at least a dozen different kinds of apples.

Artful food choices can nourish you in numerous ways. They delight your senses, give you a greater depth of wisdom and understanding about your planet, help you explore a diversity of tastes and flavors, and expand your own spiritual and physical ecology.

Also, do not limit yourself to the familiar when either buying or growing plants. There are some wonderful fruits, such as small kiwis, that are not sold commercially but are available for planting and eating.

◆

Feed your soul from the earth's own artwork.

Preparations

*We go to the grocery store and we all feel guilty
because we're not doing it from scratch.*

SANDRA LEE, WRITER

DO YOU EVER FEEL LIKE YOU SHOULD BE PREPAR-ing all your meals from scratch – like your grandmother did? Yes, freshness and ingredients are important, but there are times when preparation can include finding a more moderate and modern approach.

The Buddha promoted a middle way that navigated safely between extremes. This middle way could also be used for choosing and preparing your foods. Author and homemaker Sandra Lee, for example, believes in combining fresh and packaged ingredients. She makes the point that many good restaurants also take this approach.

Another idea? You might make some items from scratch and others with prepackaged products. Or, you could prepare certain meals from scratch and other meals prepackaged. Do not feel compelled to take an all-or-none approach.

◆

Find a happy medium in today's preparation
that suits your lifestyle.

Rituals

Grandfather,
Sacred One,
Teach us love, compassion, and honor
That we may heal the earth
And heal each other.

OJIBWAY PRAYER

 HAVE YOU EVER THOUGHT ABOUT USING A MEAL-time ritual as a way to help heal the planet? If this sounds strange, consider that you can incorporate almost any idea into your personal mealtime ritual or blessing. Many Native American traditions, for example, emphasize taking only what is needed, as well as giving back as a means of maintaining balance with nature.

How can you give back? You might take a vow during your mealtime ritual to save energy by making fewer trips to the grocery store. You could recycle when possible. Get creative and find new ways to give back.

True, many of us are blessed with plentiful resources. But that does not mean you should stop caring for the planet and those who live on it with you.

◆

Give something back to the earth
that supports your life.

Eating

*Statistics show that of those who contract the habit
of eating, very few ever survive.*

WALLACE IRWIN, WRITER

DO YOU OVEREAT? UNDEREAT? THOUGH MANY of us struggle with eating, it is very different from alcoholism or a gambling addiction. You can abstain from alcohol, for example, and survive. But you cannot abstain from eating and survive – at least not for very long.

If you struggle with eating, try this: Get a plant and put it in your kitchen – any houseplant will do. Learn to care for it, to see how fragile it is without the proper care and watering. Tended to, you can watch it grow and flourish. In the same way, nourish and care for yourself with food.

And so you must live in peace with what you are eating today, this moment. Find compassion for your natural hunger for healthy food. Find compassion for your not so healthy cravings. Accept the reality of this meal. Take a bite less (or more) than yesterday for your health.

✦

Accept today's food choices and your human
hunger with love and compassion.

Community

Kindness in giving creates love.

LAO TZU, TAOIST PHILOSOPHER

DO YOU FIND IT EASY TO OFFER FOOD TO OTHERS? Do you easily accept a meal when you are the recipient? Learning how to give to others through food is an important spiritual practice. That is because giving away food, especially food you have cooked yourself, means you are letting go of something very valuable indeed.

In Buddhism, for example, the community traditionally offers food to the monks. Since the monks cannot accept food otherwise, this giving is critical to their survival.

Personally, I can remember being offered food when I was a monk. This act of giving and love greatly humbled me. At that moment, I awakened to the connection between all persons. As independent as we think we are, we really need others to survive. It was a powerful lesson of how giving and love go together.

✦

Give some food away today
as an expression of love.

Departure

*The void gives you many choices
and new possibilities.*

SANAYA ROMAN, *Spiritual Growth*

WHEN YOU EXIT THE DINNER TABLE, DOES YOUR stomach often feel bloated and heavy? Or light but satisfied? How you feel can be a clue about whether you ate too much. Sometimes, overeating and the feeling of a filled up stomach can become a habit.

Here is a good after-meal practice to help you experience a new way to feel "full." Find a comfortable seat and settle into your normal breathing pattern. Feel the amount of breath that you inhale. Some breaths are deeper than others, but find your normal, average breath.

Experience how each breath gives you enough air, naturally, without effort. Now take one very deep, long breath, filling your belly and chest. Hold it until it becomes uncomfortable! Exhale (thankfully).

Imagine if you took every breath until you had no more space in your lungs. When you eat, breathe, and live, try to leave space for something more.

◆

Reflect on how leaving space (in your lungs
and stomach) can be natural, effortless.

Entry

The man who runs away will fight again.

MENANDER, GREEK PLAYWRIGHT

DO YOU EVER RUN AWAY FROM FOOD – EITHER from a particular food or in general? Sooner or later, however, there will be another meal, another piece of chocolate cake, another temptation. If you run from food today, you will eventually have to "fight again."

Think how much energy you expend in this emotional tug of war between avoid-shouldn't-won't and want-should-will.

Once while fasting in the monastery, for example, I was tempted by a chocolate bar. There was a dramatic mental struggle over this chocolate bar, until I simply observed the volley of emotions. I did not repress my thoughts or blame myself, but gave them space and just watched the drama. With that, I let my desire and awareness coexist in peace, and the desire soon evaporated.

Be aware of your struggle. Accept and observe that you have both skillful and unskillful thoughts.

+

Can you find tolerance and acceptance
for the unskillful thoughts, the one-sided
thoughts about food?

Choices

*If I'm feeling really radical, I'll get an
Earl Grey tea, milk, extra sweet.*

SCOTT SCHAFFER, WRITER

DO YOU HAVE A MORNING FOOD HABIT? How long has your current habit been active? Do you find convenient excuses for sticking with it? Personally, I used to have a muffin and a coffee every morning. I still remember my surprise when I learned that caffeine stays in the body for up to thirty-six hours.

The problem with any long-held food habit is that it can lead to addictive behavior, as well as blocking out other healthy variations. One benefit of breaking a routine, as I learned, is to witness the real strength of your habit.

Naturally, you will need to find a healthy substitute that nourishes your spirit. In the case of coffee, there are many decaffeinated teas available. Green tea, for example, has been shown to have several health benefits, including lowering high blood pressure and preventing cancer. In fact, it is an ancient Chinese belief that green tea has many healing properties.

◆

For one meal or snack, alter your eating
routines for beneficial health.

Preparations

*A baker is like an abbot, who serves as a guide
and guardian of the souls in his charge. . . . Simply
stated, the more nurturing a dough receives from
start to finish, the better the bread.*

BROTHER PETER REINHART,
Brother Juniper's Bread Book

 AS BROTHER REINHART WRITES, YOU ARE THE abbot of your kitchen. Sounds impressive, doesn't it? Now that you have this important role, however, how will you go about making your kitchen and home a place where food and cooking is nurtured from start to finish?

One way is to create a sense of order in your kitchen workspace. Surely, no abbot would want a messy kitchen! Store away those utensils that you do not need. Put away that coffee maker and other appliances that are normally reserved for when you have guests. Clear out the space so that what remains is uncluttered and un-encumbered.

In this way, you are the guardian of your kitchen and the guardian of mindfulness.

Unclutter your kitchen to leave room for creating the meal.

◆

Be the abbot of your kitchen space.

Rituals

*The drum is often the only instrument
used in our sacred rites.*

BLACK ELK, HOLY MAN OF THE SIOUX

DO YOU HAVE A SACRED OR SPECIAL OBJECT THAT helps to sanctify your mealtime? This can make your mealtime rich with meaning. And, as Native American medicine man Black Elk suggests, you do not need to make your rite or blessing complex.

Even a simple object will do. It will be sacred and holy so long as it has some deeper meaning for you. Black Elk's sacred drum, for example, represents the heartbeat of the universe. In many traditions, a candle represents bringing light into the home and heart.

There are many different kinds of sacred objects that you can add to your current mealtime blessing. Whether it is a crystal, candle, or photo – especially of a loved one who has passed on – try to place it in a location where it becomes part of your sacred meal. Let it inspire you (even silently) as you observe your mealtime blessing.

◆

Discover a sacred object to enrich
your mealtime blessing.

Eating

I can resist everything except temptation.

OSCAR WILDE

WHAT FOODS WOULD BE PICTURED AT THE POST office on your "ten most tempting foods" poster? Rather than let these foods have hidden power over you, you can choose to extinguish the temptation.

Wait until you are not hungry before trying this experiment! Take one small, mindful spoonful or bite of your tempting food without trying to resist it at all. You are simply conducting an experiment to concentrate on sensations of taste, smell, texture, and the energy component of the food.

Chew a minimum of twenty-five times until the food in your mouth becomes liquid and the flavor is exhausted. Observe your desire for the food (pleasant, unpleasant, or neutral) without becoming attached. Take ten mindful breaths between bites. Take as many bites as necessary to simply gain insight into your sensations and thoughts about why this food tempts you, not to derive any special pleasure. When you feel like you have more insight, end the experiment.

◆

Experience that even tempting food
is just energy to your body that receives
nourishment.

Community

Come, for today is for us a day of festival;
Henceforward joy and pleasure are on the increase

. . .

Who is there in this world like our Friend?
Who has seen such a festival in a hundred cycles?
Earth and heaven are filled with sugar;
In every direction sugarcane has sprouted.

RUMI, PERSIAN POET

HOW HAS YOUR EATING CYCLE MATURED AS YOU approach or grow into adulthood? As an adult do you find that your experience with food becomes like a harvest that is more readily enjoyed with others?

Seasonally, this is the time of year – usually June 21 or 22 – when the summer solstice occurs. The beginning of summer is marked by the longest day of the year. This represents a time of warmth from the sun and lots of growing activity in the fields.

This season can also be a very good time to warm up and develop your friendships over food. Summer is a time to be outside, to picnic, and to celebrate. It is a time to be around others at outdoor farmer's markets and fairs where food and music abound. Set aside the time to experience bliss with others during this season of growth.

◆

Experience the sweetness and warmth of
friendship that sprouts in your summer season.

Departure

With a bowl of tea, peace can truly spread.

SOSHITSU SEN XV, *Tea Life, Tea Mind*

HAVE YOU EVER NOTICED THE SHIFT IN CONVER-sation when the meal is over and the waiter or host asks if anyone would like coffee or tea? Even if you are eating alone, can you feel the subtle change that occurs when you settle into your favorite chair for an after-meal cup of tea (coffee, water, soda)?

You can use this moment to create a transitional period of peace and composure for yourself or others. It is as if the pressure is off. Hunger has been filled, and now you can relax and just be yourself.

If after-dinner magic has eluded you, try this: Admire and experience your drink as you would any beautiful thing in nature. Then, experience your guests in the same way, hearing their words without judgment, but with wonder at the intelligence we all possess.

◆

Be receptive to the natural beauty of tea,
your surroundings, and guests after dinner.

Entry

It must be hard to be hungry when
food is plentiful!

GITA MENTA

DO YOU EXPERIENCE UNSETTLING EMOTIONS AND anxious feelings more acutely before you eat? Food takes on a different significance as you approach mealtime. Fortunately, being mindful of your emotions can moderate and heal your approach to eating. The key to moderating mealtime emotions is knowing that they are temporary, like a summer rain.

Say, for example, that you approach lunchtime feeling extreme anxiety because you fear gaining weight. Maybe you looked in the mirror before lunch and were frightened by the loud voice that said, "You look fat."

Who is that voice? Is it you, or is it just a sliver of who you are? In truth, the real you has a richness and depth of experience. This frightened voice – although loud and demanding – is merely distracting you from the successful you who has conquered many life fears and has a history of eating many healthy foods.

♦

Who is the successful, authentic you?

Choices

Dietary systems based on virtual models of the
human body all too often lead to hopeless conflicts.

DON GERRARD, *One Bowl*

IS IT POSSIBLE FOR ANY ONE DIETARY SYSTEM to fit your unique human body? What do you think? Or will modifications and adaptations need to be made?

Diets assume that your body works just like every other body. Feed it X, Y, and Z, and you will always get the same results. But if you and a friend have ever been on the same diet, then you know that it does not work out that way.

Your body reflects a complex, interrelated system that includes your unique mix of genetics, allergies, hormones, desires, appetite, mood, emotions, physical makeup, and much more. Finding out what foods or dietary system is best for you takes time. And it will most certainly need adaptation.

Fitting your body into a one-size-fits-all diet can be like forcing your car to run on something other than gasoline.

◆

Examine and reflect on your body's
real dietary needs.

Preparations

At the center of a life based on harmony, respect,
purity, and tranquility is that inner peace that
results from accepting one's limits and finding
satisfaction within the incomplete.

Soshitsu Sen XV, *Tea Life, Tea Mind*

Are you a perfectionist around the kitchen? Do you get upset when the fish is overcooked, the asparagus comes out limp, and the barbecue gets charred? Who takes the blame?

No one is born a genius chef, knowing how to cook and prepare a meal. If you are like most people, you learn how to cook by trial and error.

There was a time, for example, when a friend and I tried to make the perfect deep-dish pizza. We experimented with different pizza pans, dough, toppings, and cheese. But we never could recreate that deep-dish Chicago pizza that we loved. Still, it was pretty good, and we had a couple of fun pizza parties that made our quest worthwhile.

Do not let perfection stop you from enjoying the process of preparation.

◆

Cook what you can – even if
it is out of the can!

Rituals

To Eskimos rubbing noses is a friendship ritual.

HUSTON SMITH, *The World's Religions*

 DO YOU HAVE A MEALTIME RITUAL THAT IS comfortable for you? Remember that rituals serve as more than just blessings. Any custom that you create around your mealtime can serve as a kind of ritual.

One common ritual for people – whether single or living with others – is to watch a familiar TV show at mealtime. Although mindfulness is best practiced by focusing on your meal, you may want to continue with your current custom if a TV program helps you feel relaxed and cheerful.

However, stay mindful of your meal and your breath. If you find that TV encourages unskillful and mindless eating, find another ritual to replace it right away! There are other rituals you can adopt, such as reading a book or scripture (from any tradition), listening to music, or just being silent and mindful with your meal.

◆

Become aware of your ritual and be willing
to vary it from time to time.

Eating

*If this is coffee, please bring me some tea; but if
this is tea, please bring me some coffee.*

ABRAHAM LINCOLN

HAVE YOU EVER BEEN UNHAPPY WITH YOUR FOOD selection or the amount of food on your plate (too much or too little)? Mealtime expectations can set you up for a fall. When that happens, how well do you adapt? Do you let discomfort with your food sour the rest of your meal?

When the portion size, quality, or something else is not what you expect, you have a choice. You can observe your emotions and thoughts, or you can let them spoil your meal. Or you could do as Abraham Lincoln did and request something else – although this may not always be an option. Fortunately, however, you are free to change your feelings.

Letting go of your disappointment does not mean that you like the bad food or poor service. But it does mean that you are accepting and tolerant of the situation.

◆

Let go of expectations and
adapt to the meal before you.

Community

*The best way to cheer yourself up
is to cheer somebody else up.*

MARK TWAIN

MEALTIME LAUGHTER IS OFTEN CONTAGIOUS. Personally, I can remember more than one occasion where laughter and joy were what made the meal memorable.

One of the best ways to promote a cheerful dinner table is to give everyone a voice. By that, I mean listen to those who speak. Give those with whom you share mealtime an opportunity to express what is on their minds and in their hearts.

If you have ever been criticized at the dinner table, then you know the lump in your stomach is as much the undigested emotion as the food. On the other hand, respect and dignity lay the foundation for dialogue and laughter. You can also formalize the sharing of stories around the table by giving everyone a turn to say something.

Even if you are alone, you can reflect on the story of your life today.

♦

Listen with respect and share
your story at today's meal.

Departure

Life can only be understood backwards,
but it must be lived forwards.

SØREN KIRKEGAARD, DANISH PHILOSOPHER

IT IS A PARADOX THAT YOUR MIND CAN HOLD ON to that last meal while you are moving forward in time and space. Since life must be lived in the present moment, the choice to let go of the past makes good sense.

Still, if you have trouble releasing the emotions surrounding mindless eating, you can always play events in reverse motion. Playing them in reverse may help you discover the intense feelings that you tried to bury or forget with food.

Use slow, reverse motion to back up one moment at a time until you reach the beginning of the meal. Observe and identify those moments where you lost mindful eating. Note the situation in detail, and replay the scene with a more beneficial intention and choice. Once your new choice is clear, you can move forward to the present with a joyful heart.

◆

Replay in reverse a mindless meal.
Make new mindful choices and do not
dwell on the past.

Entry

*I love food. Food movies, food novels, food just-
about-anything. . . . I like to eat, too, but regarding
food, really, it's the imagined pleasures to come
I particularly go for.*

BEVERLY LOWRY, AUTHOR

HAVE YOU EVER BEEN ELATED JUST BY IMAGINING your upcoming mealtime pleasures? Do your food fantasies exceed your actual experience with food and eating?

Some excitement around food is normal. However, food emotions can also lead to unhealthy or obsessive eating habits. For this reason, eating mindfully means even becoming aware of the excitement and fantasies you may have about food.

With mindful awareness you can go deeper and explore the why beneath your emotions. For example, in his classic book *On the Road*, author Jack Kerouac writes repeatedly of his favorite food as he travels across the United States. You can sense his excitement as he writes, "I ate apple pie and ice cream – it was getting better as I got deeper into Iowa, the pie bigger, the ice cream richer." But Kerouac does not understand, as we must, what emotional hunger or need drives his fantasy and desire.

◆

What inner hunger is beneath
the food you desire?

Choices

*If you think about it, eating is a process of
possession . . . of taking that which is not you and
receiving it within your boundaries.*

Don Gerrard, *One Bowl*

 How mindful are you about the food you receive "within your boundaries"? Do you eat what is put in front of you, without discrimination? Or are your boundaries highly protected by your own "eat" and "do not eat" lists? People who are lactose-intolerant, for example, get immediate feedback about necessary food boundaries.

The moment you put something into your mouth, you permit that substance to mix with your physical and energy bodies. This takes on significance when you realize that 34 percent of corn, 75 percent of soy products, and 15 percent of canola oil are genetically modified (GM). What is more, GM foods are increasing in number.

GM information is on some labeling. I believe it should be present on all food labeling, since long-term effects are not really known. So be mindful of your boundaries.

✦

Take responsibility for what you put
into your mouth this meal.

Preparations

Do not peek. Do not touch. Do not taste.

BILL COSBY, *The Cosby Show*

WHEN CLIFF HUXTABLE MADE CHILI, HE WENT to extremes to make sure that no one would discover the ingredients. Do you share your preparation secrets with others? Or do you keep everyone out of your kitchen during preparation time?

I find that sharing recipes and preparation secrets is another way of using food to practice love, giving, and kindness. I will never forget the time I met the man who initially developed Chicago stuffed pizza. And when I told him how much I loved his creation, he gave me his prized recipe right then and there, letting me write it down on a paper place setting!

If you have not done so, I suggest you share your preparations as you share the food you make. Here is another way of not holding on so tightly to food.

◆

Bring loved ones into your kitchen and share
preparation with those who are interested.

Rituals

*Be still and know that I am with you, says the
Lord. Be still and know I am you, says the Tao.*
MARTIN PALMER, BRITISH RELIGIOUS AUTHORITY

HAVE YOU EVER FOUND STILLNESS AT YOUR MEAL?
Have you found an inner calm where the voices of blame,
shame, and expectation grow silent and quiet? Finding stillness
through ritual blessing is a special feeling that unites you with each
bite of your meal. It is a special feeling of oneness that you cannot
quickly forget.

This place of stillness really exists. As you sit down at your table,
begin by experiencing mindful breathing. Inhale as you mentally
say, "Create a breath." Then say, "End a breath," as you exhale. Let
this rhythm still your body. Fill your belly (diaphragm) with each
life-giving breath. Settle into a slow breathing that you can continue as you eat.

Now, recite your ritual blessing (the one above or another) that
states your deep intention to be still with the divine presence around
and within you (and around and within your food).

◆

Experience the ultimate freedom
of stillness and quiet.

Eating

Never eat more than you can lift.

MISS PIGGY, MUPPET PUPPET CHARACTER

WHEN YOUR EYES ARE BIGGER THAN YOUR APpetite, do you eat all the food on your plate even if it is more than you need? Restaurants are notorious for large portions. If you are in need of portion control, this can help:

Whenever I want more control over my portions, I adapt what I learned in the monastery. I start with an empty plate. Then I take only the amount of food from the "serving" plate that I want. When I'm done, I always have the option of adding a little more food onto my plate.

Start with an empty plate, whether you eat alone or with others. You can easily do this at a restaurant by asking for an extra plate. This way, you are in control of the amount of food on your plate and can take home the "serving" plate leftovers.

◆

Control today's portions with an extra plate.

Community

A smiling face is half the meal.

LATVIAN PROVERB

ARE YOU POSSESSIVE OF YOUR FOOD? DO YOU hate it when someone asks for a taste or a bite of your meal? Or do you willingly share your meal (or dessert) with others?

It is easy to become possessive of food. Observe your own family when it comes to sharing food. Often, possessiveness is related to the idea of scarcity. When you were growing up, was food ever scarce in your home? Even stinginess from the heart can create an unwillingness to let go and give food. If you recognize this trait in yourself, you can make a conscious effort to open up.

In the movie *Thunderheart*, for example, there's an inspired moment when a shaman hands an apple to an FBI agent, who takes a big bite. Then the shaman motions for him to leave the rest of the apple on a nearby pie plate as an offering to spirit.

At today's meal, give a portion of your meal to a neighbor or just feed the birds with an extra piece of bread. As you become less possessive about food, you will be more relaxed around it.

◆

Observe how possessive you are
with food. Let go a little.

Departure

Money won't buy you happiness, but
happiness won't buy you groceries.

ANONYMOUS

HAVE YOU EVER LEFT A MEAL THINKING THAT because you had eaten a lot of food that you "got your money's worth"? Certainly, the value of the food on your plate can be examined from different perspectives. But if you often "value" food according to how much you can eat per dollar spent, then you may actually be shortchanging yourself.

One temptation is to eat as much as possible to get more for your money. Eating at all-you-can-eat buffets can be challenging for this very reason. Another temptation is to try as many different dishes as possible because it costs no extra. Either way, bingeing is not beneficial to your emotional, physical, and spiritual well-being.

When you find yourself falling into these scenarios, take as many mindful breaths as you need to bring you back to your intention to eat mindfully, skillfully, and beneficially.

◆

Shift from the meal's monetary value to its
mindfulness value and beneficial value.

Entry

*There lies before us, if we choose, continued
progress in happiness, knowledge, and wisdom. . . .
Remember your humanity and forget the rest.*

ALBERT EINSTEIN

IS SOMETHING EATING YOU AS YOU APPROACH mealtime? Anger and negative emotions can cause physical upset through ulcers, migraines, and a host of other problems. Emotions can also change your food choices, causing you to eat heavier foods to block them out or making you lose your appetite altogether.

If emotions make it difficult for you to eat without feeling nervous and stressed out, then you need to do as Einstein said: "Remember your humanity and forget the rest."

If you cannot do this completely, you can still practice it a little. Before mealtime, say, "Let me forgive for the moment so that I may eat and be nourished without unhealthy emotions getting in the way."

If you are not ready to forgive, you can simply accept things the way they are. This does not mean you like them, but you can suspend your emotions long enough to enjoy your meal.

✦

You don't have to forgive today, but reflect
on how eating without negative emotion
heals your body, mind, and spirit.

Choices

There's small choice in rotten apples.

WILLIAM SHAKESPEARE, *Taming of the Shrew*

 MORE AND MORE OF US ARE EATING OUT AT restaurants. How often do you eat out? In general, restaurant meals are higher in calories. In all, this contributes to the fact that the average American now eats 500 more calories a day than we did just twenty-five years ago. Add that up for a year and the total is astounding.

Sure, there are good restaurants out there serving lighter, healthier fare. But how often do you ask, for example, at every restaurant, what kind of oil they use when cooking? The point here is not to avoid restaurant eating. Neither is it to become frightened about your calorie count.

This is all about your choices. What are your habitual restaurant choices? What else is available for you? Seek out the "fresh apples" where and when you can.

◆

Be mindful of your restaurant choices today.

Preparations

*The greatest mistake you can make in life is to be
continually fearing you will make one.*

ELBERT HUBBARD, AUTHOR

GIVING UP HOPE OF MAKING A FANTASTIC MEAL does not mean that you do not try. But you realize that relinquishing the goal gives you the freedom to make the preparation experience more joyful.

Does fear ever stop you from trying a new recipe? Do you ever want to make a special dish but do not because it seems too difficult?

Years ago while taking a professional chef's class, for example, I had to make puff pastry. I knew that my finished product would be judged and tasted by the entire class – not to mention my highly accomplished chef instructor. Still, I forged ahead with abandonment, rolling out the dough into thin layers, folding and chilling it, then rolling it out again.

You too can let go of any goal beforehand and fully enjoy the experience – independent of judging by yourself or others.

◆

Acknowledge your fear and go ahead
anyway. Let the experience be your friend.

Rituals

I vow to practice mindful breathing and smiling,
looking deeply into all things.

THICH NHAT HANH

IF YOU COMMIT TO THIS MEALTIME VOW – EVEN for a day – it can alter the way you eat. Remember that you do not have to change all your eating habits today. Even a little change is a good one.

Always settle in to your meal with an inviting breath. Mindfulness is focus, so put your awareness on your breath and see if you can keep it there during your meal. There will be times when you forget, but as you eat, see if you can keep 10 to 25 percent of your attention focused on your breath. Make a point of taking at least one conscious breath between bites. This is important.

Then, use the rest of your attention to look deeply into the nature of the food and your thoughts as you eat. Whatever you experience is a success.

◆

Focus on breathing while you eat.

Eating

The secret of staying young is to live honestly,
eat slowly, and lie about your age.
LUCILLE BALL

DO YOU EAT SLOWLY AND DELIBERATELY? DO YOU savor each bite or gulp it down? Eating slowly may, in fact, help you discover the real taste of food. You may find that a food tastes better (or worse) when you really taste it.

I know a man who learned mindful eating with olives – a food he regularly ate. During his mindful eating exercise he learned – to his surprise and chagrin – that he disliked the flavor. He has not eaten an olive since.

Slowing down with each bite has another benefit. It takes about fifteen or twenty minutes for the body to register the feeling of fullness after eating. If you eat quickly, you can overeat before you ever feel satiated.

Take deliberate bites, chew your food until it softens into liquid – thereby aiding digestion. Examine all your sensations.

◆

Savor your meal by slowing down
and really tasting it in detail.

Community

*There's somebody at every dinner party
who eats all the celery.*

KIN HUBBARD, AUTHOR

DO YOU GET ANXIOUS OR IMPATIENT IN A CAFE-
teria line, afraid that your favorite dish will be scoffed up?
Or do you feel greed well up in you when the serving tray is passed
to you at a communal meal? Do you feel that you may not get
enough food to eat?

Feelings of greed and impatience around food are no reason to
blame oneself for being selfish. It is enough to notice your feelings.
When you feel these thoughts, just silently repeat "greed, greed" or
"impatience, impatience" to yourself. By labeling your thoughts,
you separate them from you. This also lets you witness how each
thought begins and ends.

Now, take a mindful breath. When your time comes to take
food, have compassion for the part of you that acts out of a feeling
of scarcity and greed.

◆

Label your thoughts of greed
or impatience with food.

Departure

*It's okay to be fat. So you're fat. Just be fat
and shut up about it.*

ROSEANNE BARR

IF YOU THINK YOUR BODY WEIGHT IS HEAVY, thin, or in between, how does it make you feel? I do not mean in relation to others – although no one wants to be judged. Neither do I refer to potential health issues raised by your weight. The question here is simply this: Deep down inside, how do you feel about your weight?

I know of a true story of a young boy who was always the heaviest in his class at school. He felt bad about this until one day when he had an epiphany. He came home excited and told his mom, "Other boys are just taller than me. I am just wider than them."

That was it!

Everyone can learn from the amazing wisdom of this young boy. Even though you may still want to change your body weight for health reasons, you do not need to let your body define who you are as a person.

✦

How do you feel about your body? What is
your wisdom about this?

Entry

*There is small danger of being starved
in our land of plenty; but the danger of
being stuffed is imminent.*

SARAH JOSEPHA HALE,
NINETEENTH-CENTURY WRITER

WHEN YOU APPROACH TODAY'S MEAL, WHAT IS your imminent danger? Can you anticipate what foods, habits, or eating styles can derail your mindful eating?

The advantage of being mindful as you enter a meal is that it prepares you for what is to come. When you drive, for example, don't you look ahead to avoid cars that might unexpectedly pull into your lane? Likewise, mindful entry to mealtime gives you the same protection against "eating accidents." Fortunately, you have a built-in insurance policy for this – your mindfulness.

Anticipate the foods you expect to see at the location where you will have your meal. Do this when you go to the grocery store, too. By knowing the temptations you will face, you do not have to automatically react to the cravings and desires that arise. Instead, you can observe them with mindfulness.

◆

Use mindfulness to anticipate and
strengthen you as you approach your meal.

Choices

I wish my ulcers and I could get together
on a mutually satisfactory diet.
IRVIN S. COBB, AUTHOR

 DO YOU HAVE HEALTH PROBLEMS THAT ARE RE-lated to your eating and diet? Ulcers, heartburn, high cholesterol, and indigestion are signs that your diet, emotional eating style, and lifestyle may need adjustment.

I know a man who had health problems relating to his diet. His doctor gave him a new eating and exercise regimen. Instead of following the doctor's advice, he had another solution: Find a new doctor. Unfortunately, that kind of mindless approach did not make his problems go away.

As you age, you may need a more mindful diet for optimal health and well-being. In making changes, you can take the glass half-empty or glass half-full approach. Instead of focusing on what you are giving up, look at what you are gaining. This can be new foods, a more active lifestyle, and a better quality of life from day to day.

◆

Reflect on how your diet "fits" with your
body and health needs. Today, make one
small dietary change to benefit you.

Preparations

*A recipe is only a theme, which an intelligent cook
can play each time with a variation.*

MADAME BENOIT, CANADIAN COOKBOOK AUTHOR

DO YOU COOK OR PREPARE THE SAME MEAL OVER and over to save time? Yes, it is easy to shop and cook when you know exactly what foods you like, without having to expend any extra energy or emotion. However, eating the same food over and over may not give you the variety your body needs. In fact, it may keep you emotionally stuck in your eating patterns.

One simple answer may be to vary the dishes you normally prepare. Since you already have certain dishes that you prefer, adding a new side dish or new ingredient – even to a TV dinner – can help you discover new tastes and nutrients. Look at all the variations that exist, for example, for something like a salad. You can transform your signature salad into a caesar salad, chef salad, cobb salad, bean salad, tomato salad, tuna salad, egg salad, and so on.

◆

Be creative with preparation by using a
variation on your mealtime theme.

Rituals

*Now we will feel no rain, for each of us will be
shelter for the other.
Now we will feel no cold, for each of us will be
warmth for the other.
Now there is no more loneliness, for each of us will
be companion to the other.*

APACHE WEDDING BLESSING

HAVE YOU EVER SAT DOWN TO A MEAL FEELING the need for support and encouragement? If you are exhausted from your daily routine, weary from your struggle with food and diet, then use this blessing.

You do not need to endure your food struggle alone. This mealtime blessing can help you rest in the web of being that surrounds you. It brings you closer to others by acknowledging your need for shelter, warmth, food, and companionship that is common to all beings.

Let this blessing open you to the healing and help that others are willing to provide for you. Personally, I know there are enlightened registered dietitians, nutritionists, and counselors who specialize in this area. I consider them angels here on Earth. Overcome your fear and seek them out.

✦

Open to receiving companionship, warmth,
healing, and shelter from your personal storms.

Eating

Without attention, the human sense of wonder
and the holy will stir occasionally, but to become
a steady flame it must be tended.

HUSTON SMITH, *The World's Religions*

How often do you tend your flame of mindfulness at mealtime? This is one of the great challenges of eating. It is all too easy to drift back to mindlessness where the sense cravings and emotions can take control. Mealtime can be a time of escapism, or it can be a time to be in the moment. Today's meal is a chance to be awake instead of sleepwalking through life.

Tending the flame requires two things: enthusiasm and effort. Hopefully, these meditations inspire you and fire up your enthusiasm. But to keep the enthusiasm you need the effort to stay on the path daily.

There are five basic obstacles to effort that can lead to mindless eating. These include food cravings and desires, unhealthy emotions and focusing on negativity, sleepiness and fatigue, anxiety and restlessness, and doubt. Be mindful of when they appear.

◆

For now, simply watch for the five
obstacles to effort. When they get in the way,
simply note them as "desire, desire" and
"fatigue, fatigue," and so on.

Community

*Often I think the main point of life is having
something to talk about at dinner.*

JERRY HALL, MODEL

IS IT IMPORTANT FOR YOU TO HAVE SOMETHING
to talk about at dinner? You can take it a step further. The
ancient Christian prayer practice of *lectio divina*, or sacred reading,
gives you – either alone or as a group – the opportunity to feel divine presence at mealtime.

Originally, *lectio divina* was practiced by the desert monks of
Egypt in the second and third centuries. Today it is being rediscovered. The idea is to read out loud a short passage of scripture,
a poem, or other meaningful writing over and over until the presence of the divine is revealed. If a particular word or phrase jumps
out at you, narrow your focus to read that sentence over and over.

Speak softly, and listen to the words come back to you as if this
was something you could have written. The experience is something received, rather than taken. Let whatever you feel – boredom, love, frustration, anger, grace – be your experience of the
divine at this moment. (The reading usually lasts twenty-five to
forty minutes.)

◆

Set the intention to experience the divine at
mealtime, then begin your reading.

Departure

*I would like to find a stew that will give
me heartburn immediately, instead of at
three o'clock in the morning.*

JOHN BARRYMORE

DO YOUR CURRENT FOOD CHOICES LEAVE YOU WANT-
ing fewer side effects and discomforts? Is temporary food
pleasure worth discomfort or even long-term health problems?

You need to be mindful and very honest with yourself. Depending on your family history, for example, your diet may make
you susceptible to diabetes and other serious conditions. In some
cases, these health problems can be managed by proper diet.

When you know you have just eaten a meal that risks your
health, how do you feel afterward? Do you worry about it, deny it,
or rationalize it? Mindfulness means taking responsibility for your
physical and mental feelings after your meal. Listen to your body
after the meal, and it will tell you the truth about your eating.

◆

Be honest about the side effects
of risky eating.

Entry

When ordering lunch the big executives
are just as indecisive as the rest of us.

WILLIAM FEATHER, AUTHOR

ARE YOU INDECISIVE AS YOU APPROACH MEALTIME? If so, then welcome to this very inclusive club. Most people do not know what they want until they step into the kitchen or restaurant. Ancestrally speaking, there is probably a good reason why most people like to forage for their food!

Fortunately, you can transform indecision into clarity by having guidelines for your upcoming meal. If you follow a dietary plan, then you probably have guidelines in place. If not, take a mindful breath and scan your body. Sense the kind of food that you need for energy and well-being. You can also scan the items on a restaurant menu. As you do so, imagine the purity and energy of this food being absorbed into your cells and consciousness.

At the same time, watch for the cravings and emotional desires related to your meal. If you practice this enough, you will eventually be able to separate what your body needs from what your emotions crave.

◆

Before you enter today's meal, scan your
body for the food you need.

Choices

*The mind that does not know is in a state of
learning . . . then there is a movement of flexibility,
of harmony, because the mind does not know.*

KRISHNAMURTI, *On Relationship*

DO YOU DECIDE WHAT YOU WANT TO EAT AT THE last moment? Many weight-loss diets do not give you this freedom and spontaneity.

Whenever you undertake any restrictive weight-loss diet, you may lose the flexibility to create a healthy harmony between food and your body. Still, I have on rare occasion tried a specific diet just to break my old eating patterns and try new food combinations. Whenever I do this, however, I pay very close attention to how I feel and how my body reacts.

Do not feel bound by a diet's constraints if you feel weak or sick. It is okay to give yourself permission to undertake a new approach to eating, so long as you retain the right to choose and adapt. To become a slave to any diet is to lose your free will!

◆

Maintain your mindful eating choices
with flexibility and freedom.

Preparations

Even the finest of cookbooks is no substitute
for the poorest of dinners.
ALDOUS HUXLEY

YOU CANNOT EAT A COOKBOOK. (THERE ARE NONE edible that I know of.) And so, it is enough that you do your best to prepare a meal and appreciate the finished product. Sometimes, this means accepting those times that you may not have the best-quality meat, cooking pot, or variety of spices.

Acceptance is an important seasoning for preparation and cooking. With mindful acceptance, your completed meal is free of bitterness, regret, and expectation. For Buddhist monks in Thailand, Burma, and Laos, for example, preparation consists of walking door-to-door asking for food. In their one bowl go all types of food – rice, fish, homemade stew, noodles, even Coca-Cola! Then, it is brought back to the monastery and mixed together.

Your preparation is sacred, whether you cook steak, beans, macaroni, or a TV dinner. Even the simplest meal is a gift when stirred with acceptance.

◆

Prepare with acceptance and gratitude;
have gratitude for what you prepare.

Rituals

*May the passions of lust, anger, greed, pride and
attachment depart from me. O Lord, I come to
seek Thy shelter: Bless me with thy grace.*

SACRED SONG OF THE SIKHS

HOW STRONG ARE YOUR EMOTIONS AT MEALTIME?
Do you feel swept up in the drama of the day? Do you watch
the news while eating, all the while feeling your blood pressure boil?
If so, then you may want to consider using a ritual blessing similar
to the one above.

A mealtime ritual blessing like the Sacred Song of the Sikhs is
a touchstone for revealing and reveling in the deeper meaning of
your meal. In another sense, this mealtime ritual blessing directly
connects you to the spiritual aspect of your meal.

That aspect may be nonattachment to food, as well as finding
peace and the grace of God at mealtime. Let yourself rest in the
wisdom of this ritual blessing as you say it. Take a mindful, grateful breath afterward as you let the meaning seep into your innermost being. Amen.

◆

Let this blessing free you from passions that
disrupt your mealtime grace and peace.

Eating

Surrender is inner acceptance of what is
without any reservations. . . . Surrender does
not transform what is, at least not directly.
Surrender transforms you.

ECKHART TOLLE, *The Power of Now*

DO YOU EVER FEEL THE URGE TO BINGE, OVEREAT, or engage in other disordered eating? Instead of waging a battle against the impulse, can you accept that the voice you hear at this moment is one part of you? Can you find peace with the voice through acceptance and awareness of it?

Where is the fight taking place? Who is engaged in this battle, anyway? There is no fight if you decide to just watch like a bystander. By hearing your voice of despair, you can surrender to it and accept its presence. But that does not mean you need to submit to it by following through with a destructive action.

If you do lose mindfulness and submit to your urge, you can compassionately return to the inner acceptance of your action – knowing that you are still a whole person, a valuable person.

◆

Inner surrender and acceptance
builds up strength over time.

Community

Isn't there any other part of the matzo you can eat?

MARILYN MONROE

WHAT DO YOU EAT WHEN INVITED TO SOMEONE'S home? Do you request special food? Do you let food dictate your attendance at parties? Or do you wish, like Marilyn Monroe, that you had known what was being served before being stuck with just "matzo."

Recently, my wife and I went to dinner with some new friends. Someone commented, "We definitely have to get together again. We like the same foods!" Shared food likes can definitely affect how you relate to others at mealtime. It may even limit the meals you eat with others.

When people come to my home, I often ask if they have any special requests. But when I am invited out, I prefer to follow in the footsteps of those like Buddha and Jesus, who ate what foods were offered.

There is no right or wrong approach here. But you can kindly and skillfully let your needs be known without judgment and opinion.

◆

How do you let others know
what food you prefer?

Departure

*Increase in strength is due not to the quantity of
nutrients with which you supply your body, but to
the quantity of what it absorbs.*

ARISTOTLE

How do you assist your body in absorbing the nutrients it needs? How do you apply Aristotle's commonsense understanding of digestion? Actually, there are several ways to approach this.

As you age, you need to be mindful of how your digestive system works. Is it more efficient with some foods and less efficient with others?

Some believe that raw fruits, for example, are best eaten between meals because they are more difficult to digest at mealtime. This may be especially true in the winter or when your body is cold. Try a mindful experiment to see how eating fruit during or after your meal changes your digestion. (Of course, check with a nutritionist or doctor before making any dietary changes.)

Use your departure from the meal to relax and give your body time to digest before you jump into an activity, especially a strenuous one.

✦

Assist your body in absorbing nutrients.

Entry

*The rhythm of life changes. Cooking must
always change with it.*

ALAIN DUCASSE, CHEF

HOW DOES THE RHYTHM OF YOUR DAY AFFECT
your eating? Whether you are very active or sedate prior to
mealtime, you can use mindful walking to establish a moderate
pace that carries forward into your meal.

For example, if you are active and restless before mealtime, then
mindful walking can slow and calm you down. And if you happen
to be sluggish, it can charge you with the focus and energy necessary for mindful eating.

Walking outside is helpful because of the fresh air and spacious
sky – especially if you've been cooped up in a building. Set the intention to lift each foot and move it forward. Observe and feel each
foot rise and move through the air. What part of your foot touches
down when you place it onto the ground? Experience each movement fully. Do this for five minutes before eating (or mindfully
walk to your meal).

◆

Set a pace for your meal with
a short mindful walk.

Choices

Sour, sweet, bitter, pungent – all must be tasted.

CHINESE PROVERB

 EVERY CULTURE HAS FOODS THAT FEATURE VAR-
ious tastes and flavors. Differences in climate and locally
grown foods probably account for many of these distinctions. Is
there a predominant flavor, or taste, in your food choices? When
was the last time, for example, that you had a food that was pungent or bitter?

Be mindful of the tastes of your foods. The American diet is
fairly aligned with sweet, salty, and sour foods. But there are not
too many bitter or pungent foods, with the exception of some
southern and regional cooking. Still, you can experience the bliss of
these other flavors by eating at different ethnic restaurants. Thai,
Chinese, Indian, and Persian cuisine are filled with spices that give
food all flavors.

You may decide to experiment by adding some of these flavors
to your own meals.

◆

Try a food flavor that is out of your "normal"
range, such as sour, bitter, or pungent.

Preparations

An army marches on its stomach.

NAPOLEON

DO YOUR MEALTIME PREPARATIONS REFLECT your body's "marching orders"? In other words, how well do your preparations anticipate your upcoming food and energy requirements?

Suppose you are going to an important morning meeting. What kind of breakfast will give you mental clarity and alertness? Or suppose you will be doing physical labor in a cold climate. What meal preparation will give you what you need to exert yourself?

In addition, you need to be mindful of how your exertion and effort prior to preparation could have an effect on what you cook right now. A stressful day, for example, might leave you wanting a really satisfying and nourishing dinner to end the day.

Be mindful of the effect of light, hearty, and heavy foods on your body. Learn which food offsets cold, heat, or fatigue, and you will be ready to march in any season or condition.

◆

Be mindful of the effects of different
foods on your ability to function under
different conditions.

Rituals

Gaia, mother of all
Foundation of all,
The oldest one. . . .
Queen of Earth
Through you
Beautiful children,
Beautiful harvests come.

ANCIENT GREEK PRAYER

 DO YOU EVER STOP TO CONSIDER THAT THE FOOD on your plate has a direct connection to the Earth? Actually, a mealtime blessing based on this idea can be traced back to the ancient Greeks, who celebrated the planet as a living entity on which you – and all of us – depend. When you acknowledge your Earth connection with such a blessing, how does it change your relationship to food?

Adding a ritual blessing like the one above can help you experience the interactive relationship that exists between you, your meal, and the care of the planet. A healthy planet means a good harvest. In turn, the Earth heals your hunger and sustains you with each bite. The next time you feel down because you think food is the enemy, use a blessing to experience how food brings you into communion with the wellness of every living thing.

✦

Say a blessing for the living planet that
provides your well-being.

Eating

Oh, the pleasure of eating my dinner alone!

CHARLES LAMB, NINETEENTH-CENTURY
ENGLISH CRITIC AND ESSAYIST

WHAT IS IT LIKE FOR YOU TO EAT ALONE? HOW different is the experience of eating alone compared to eating with others? For some, solitary dining may bring up feelings of loneliness and aloneness. For others, such as Charles Lamb, eating alone is both liberating and emancipating. It offers a chance to revel in food without being afraid of what others think about what you are eating. And, it gives those who like to dine alone a peaceful solitude free of mindless chatter that allows the experience to become sacred.

What this comes down to is your personal perspective. It is worth exploring your own biases. By looking closely at your attitudes and opinions, you do not have to let eating with or without others make you feel either sad or joyful.

Instead, you can simply accept the reality of "what is" and let the food experience take center stage. Choose to feel satisfied and fulfilled, and you will be!

◆

Observe your thoughts when eating
alone or with others. What judgments
and opinions come up? Accept these
and enjoy your meal anyway.

Community

*Offerings of food have been breaking down
barriers for centuries.*

ESTÉE LAUDER, COSMETICS MOGUL

DO YOU EVER NEGOTIATE SOMETHING OVER A breakfast, lunch, or dinner? Martha Stewart, for example, often brought along homemade baked goods and other foods to influence potential investors when making a business presentation.

You, too, can use the power of food to break through your personal eating patterns. By introducing new foods in a family, or communal setting, for instance, you negotiate new eating behaviors. Even a little taste of a new and exotic food can break your family's ingrained patterns of eating and invigorate it with new energy.

Do not underestimate the power of food to break down barriers. It may even get you or others discussing how you view change in your lives. You can introduce new food to make change less scary, even in a very subtle and gentle way.

◆

Use food to negotiate a new eating pattern
or behavior – for yourself and others.

Departure

A woman is like a teabag – only in hot water
do you realize how strong she is.

NANCY REAGAN

❋ ARE YOU MINDFUL OF WHAT YOU DRINK AFTER
eating and how it affects your digestion? Do you ever use
tea as medicine for your digestion and stirred-up emotions after a
meal? In traditional Chinese and Eastern medicine, for example,
hot water and hot herbal teas – including ginger tea – are thought
to enhance the power of your digestive juices, as well as soothe your
temperament.

Iced drinks consumed at mealtime are believed to have the opposite effect, dampening the power of digestive juices. (The Os-
teoporosis Education Project, a nonprofit research group, agrees
with this.)

A soothing cup of tea also makes a nice transition into what
comes after your meal. Some studies also show that tea may also
benefit and stimulate the immune system. Whether you are alone
or with others, you can try different teas to explore their effect on
your digestion and mood. Also, you may want to pay close attention to the effects of tea containing caffeine.

✦

Be mindful of what you drink after
your meal. Explore how tea may improve
your transition and digestion.

Entry

*A man has no better thing under the sun than to
eat, and to drink, and to be merry.*

ECCLESIASTES 8:15

WHAT IS THE FIRST THING TO "GO AWAY" IN YOUR
life when you are under pressure and stress? Do you lose
your appetite or skip meals? Do you stop eating nutritiously and
mindlessly eat junk food instead? Do you ignore your diet plan and
stop exercising? It is important to be aware of your usual behavior
under stress if you are to change it.

I know a woman, for example, whose good eating habits dis-
appeared during times of high stress. After recognizing this, she
wisely decided to do the opposite. Now, whenever she anticipates
stress she goes out of her way to prepare especially tasty and nu-
tritious meals. In this way, she skillfully counteracts the effects of
stress by practicing self-care.

Feeding yourself well is an excellent way of caring for yourself and
others.

◆

Choose a self-care eating strategy
when stressed out.

Choices

*[An herb is] the friend of physicians
and the praise of cooks.*

CHARLEMAGNE, KING OF THE FRANKS

DO YOU STICK WITH THE BASICS AND SHY AWAY from untried herbal edibles? Chances are that you have already tried many herbs, though you may not be aware of it. Some herbs can have medicinal and calming effects on your body and emotions.

When the Pilgrims ate cranberries at the first Thanksgiving celebration, for example, they made a good choice of herbs to add to their meal. The ability of cranberries to prevent urinary tract infections illustrates how nature or natural remedies developed long before pharmaceutical ones.

Do not forget garlic, which has been used as everything from a battlefield antibiotic in World War I to a natural way to reduce cholesterol and blood pressure.

Chamomile is a natural tranquilizer. If you have trouble sleeping, a cup of chamomile tea at night may calm your nerves and anxiety around food struggles. It can also be useful for soothing stomachaches and indigestion.

Be mindful of these and other helpful herbs when scanning your mealtime choices.

◆

Be mindful of herbs for meal and
after-meal benefits.

Preparations

What is food to one may be fierce poisons to others.

LUCRETIUS, ROMAN POET

WHEN YOU PREPARE MEALS, ARE YOU MINDFUL of how heating food changes it? Do you feel emotionally and physically better, for example, after eating raw vegetables as opposed to cooked ones? Or vice versa? Or is there a combination that works best for you?

The answer to any preparation method – from high heat to low heat to no heat – depends on your unique body. Proponents of raw vegetables and low-heat cooking, for example, maintain that foods lose enzymes when cooked with high heat. Advocates of high-heat cooking, on the other hand, contend that cooked food is more easily absorbed and helps the body's digestive juices.

Become more mindful of how food preparation makes you feel. Look for the middle way, and always consult with your physician and your nutritionist. Any one-size-fits-all approach could have serious consequences.

◆

Be more mindful of how cooking methods
can affect your physical and mental states.

Rituals

Blessed are You, Lord our God, Eternal One,
Who grants us life, sustains us, and
helps us to reach this day.

TRADITIONAL JEWISH BLESSING

DO YOU EVER FEEL WEARY OF YOUR INNER CONflict with food and eating? Do you sometimes feel like food is a burden and that you are losing the battle? If so, then here is a ritual blessing that brings things into focus and can help change your relationship to food.

As you say this blessing at your meal, think about the top three highlights of your life – those times when you felt blessed with joy and happiness – such as a birthday, graduation, or other event that happened to you last week, last year, or back in grade school. Think about this until you feel a sense of well-being spread through you from head to toe.

Now, reflect on the fact that without the sustaining nourishment of food in your life, that wonderful event could never have taken place. Then return to the life highlight and again bask in the feeling of joy.

◆

Reflect on life highlights made possible
through the nourishment of food.

Eating

An airline is a great place to diet.

WOLFGANG PUCK, CHEF

 DO YOU FIND THAT YOU HAVE MORE CONTROL over your eating depending on the time and place? I know a woman who eats a healthy diet during the day while taking care of her children. But in the evening she often eats compulsively until going to bed. Compulsive evening eating is not uncommon.

If your eating habits feel more compulsive at one time and place than another, then you need to become more aware of why. What event (or lack) triggers your emotional eating habit? Compulsive eating may be a way to distract you from looking more closely at your life and relationships. Or you may eat out of boredom because you are not deeply engaged in an alternate, meaningful activity.

It is also important to look at those times when you do not eat this way. At times like these, what is different in your life? Identify these strengths and use them to help you succeed with today's eating and mealtime.

◆

Succeed in your eating today by looking at
what worked for you in the past.

Community

A brook comes from the sea by way of the heavens.
It seems to be a unit which is separated from
everything else, but it is forever connected with the
heavens and the sea.

WALTER RUSSELL, *The Message of the Divine Iliad*

HAVE YOU EVER GROWN AND PICKED YOUR OWN tomatoes, potatoes, and green beans? Do you know what it feels like to eat food that you helped to grow and nurture? In many countries of the world, villagers and farming communities traditionally gather and contribute to picking the harvest. It is typical for many of them to sing as they reap the bounty of food in the fields.

Even if you live in an urban center, there are farms where you can experience the joy of picking your own fruits and vegetables. Walk between the long rows of plants, smell the soil, and kneel down to pluck a ripe tomato or cucumber from the vine. Another idea is to create your own small herb garden in a flower or window planter that receives sunlight during the day.

Remember: The food on your plate is a miracle of cooperative effort.

◆

Recognize the mutual miracle of
the harvest effort that occurs in the fields
and on your plate.

Departure

I'm the paragon of a couch potato.
I've got six couches.

BILL WAVRIN, CHEF

EVEN PROFESSIONAL CHEFS CAN HAVE PROBLEMS with their weight. Chef Bill Wavrin, for example, had problems moderating his eating due to sluggishness. Do you ever struggle with this same issue?

Sleepiness, sluggishness, or laziness right after leaving a meal can be a normal thing. But if it turns into three hours of mindlessly eating junk food on the couch, then you need to stop the pattern and energize yourself.

You can overcome sluggishness by practicing a deep-breathing exercise. Sit in a chair with your back straight. Now take a deep breath by inhaling deep into your diaphragm. Hold your breath for a count of five. Then, release the breath through your mouth. Take at least five breaths like this. This practice will build up heat and energy in your body. Do it until you feel a surge of alertness that keeps you from mindless nibbling.

Also, an after-dinner walk is an invigorating curative for sluggishness or poor digestion.

◆

Use mindful deep breathing to
regain mindfulness and overcome your
after meal sluggishness.

Entry

In two decades I've lost a total of 789 pounds.
I should be hanging from a charm bracelet.

ERMA BOMBECK, SYNDICATED COLUMNIST

DO YOU CARRY THE BATTLE SCARS OF YO-YO dieting with you into your next meal? Maintaining any diet for an extended period of time can be difficult. Diets can become boring and repetitive. Or the motivation around your diet can change.

Your next meal does not have to be another yo-yo struggle. Fortunately, your body has a biological heritage that is tens of thousands of years old! Be mindful of this built-in wisdom by listening and awakening to your needs, emotions, and inner perceptions of the food you eat.

Sometimes, problems with maintaining healthy eating are connected to an addiction to sugar or caffeine. If you feel this is the case, then you may want to find a nutritionist, dietitian, or doctor who specializes in this area. Under any circumstances, you can let go of yo-yo dieting and experience what you really need most to nourish you at today's meal.

◆

Let go of yo-yo dieting expectations at
today's meal. Be aware of food cravings and
possible addictions.

Choices

*If you wish to grow thinner, diminish
your dinner.... And never touch bread
till it's toasted – or stale.*

H. S. Leigh, poet

How strongly do you stick with your healthy food choices? Do you have excellent resolve until you walk past the ice-cream case or until a waiter waves the cheesecake beneath your nose? It is always good to remember that your present food habits are the result of similar choices made over and over again!

Making new choices begins with acceptance of your past and present choices, along with forgiveness. Forgiveness gives you a clean slate and helps you start fresh with your new choices. But there is another step in sticking to your food choices: a vow to eat differently – even if that change is a small one (like eating one less spoonful of cream).

A vow is like an extra strong commitment. Usually, vows are taken in the presence of others – or even the divine. Make your vow sacred by experiencing it in a sacred place or at a special time. Be sure to craft a vow that you can succeed at by making it realistic and achievable.

◆

Accept, forgive, and take a sacred vow to
help gain strength with your food choices.

Preparations

*True intelligence operates silently. Stillness is where
creativity and solutions to problems are found.*

ECKHART TOLLE, *Stillness Speaks*

AS YOU PREPARE A MEAL, HOW CRITICAL ARE YOU of your own creation? Do you worry excessively that others will not like it? Are you crestfallen when no one compliments your meal?

One key to preparation is to foster an attitude of openness and stillness. This also includes being open to the creativity of others. Many good chefs constantly taste their food as they cook. It is not uncommon for cooks to let others taste their food and to ask, "What's missing?"

Stillness and openness are not signs of weakness, but strength. When you take on the burden of something completely by yourself, that responsibility can be heavy. Share the responsibility of preparation with your inner creative source, your family, and others. A shared burden is lighter.

Let yourself enjoy the flow of ideas that is part of preparation.

◆

Invite stillness and openness to share in the
responsibility of preparation and tasting.

Rituals

May all beings be well, happy, and at peace.
May they be free from pain, hunger, and suffering.

TRADITIONAL BUDDHIST BLESSING

DO YOU EVER SIT DOWN TO A MEAL FILLED WITH a sense of gratitude and the desire that others could enjoy similar blessings? When you read the newspaper and look at the news, do you feel a great compassion for those who go hungry? If so, here is a prayer that can be recited at mealtime that helps you create peace at mealtime by transmitting your loving kindness to others.

This blessing acknowledges that as you eat, others are not as fortunate. Many live where there is little opportunity for health, peace, and food. You can transmit your prayers throughout your mealtime with this blessing or one like it.

With each bite you take, feel the power of this blessing spreading to others. Begin by sending the blessing to yourself and then expanding it to others: those at your table, your neighborhood, your city, your country, and finally, all countries.

✦

Share your wish for all beings to
enjoy food and happiness.

Eating

Hunger is the best sauce.

PROVERB

HOW HUNGRY DO YOU GET DURING THE DAY? Do you become even more ravenous as you start eating? The more aware that you become of your hunger, the better you can anticipate when you need food and the better you can prepare a backup plan.

Here is one good practice: Become more mindful of your hunger by describing it. What does your hunger feel like? How big is your hunger? Where is it located? Is it in your mouth, your stomach, your neck, your body, your mind? If your hunger were an animal, what kind of animal would it be?

You can experience your hunger anytime during the day, including while you eat. When you eat, you can experience your hunger during those moments when you take slow, mindful breaths between bites. As you eat more, where does your hunger go? What does it feel like as it peaks from extreme to moderate to none?

◆

Describe your feeling of hunger
at today's meal.

Community

There's a great new rice diet that
always works – you use one chopstick.
RED BUTTONS, COMEDIAN

Do YOUR FAMILY AND COMMUNITY MEALS HELP you explore the sacred side of eating? I am reminded of a story that reveals the potential of the community to tap into the spiritual.

In the story, a man has died and is given a guided tour of both heaven and hell. His guide first takes him to hell. There he sees the most incredible banquet of delectable foods and aromas. The only catch is that the people in hell can only eat by using three-foot-long chopsticks. The food can never reach their lips.

When he is taken to heaven he witnesses the identical banquet table of mouth-watering foods and desserts. And again, everyone must eat with the same three-foot-long chopsticks.

"I don't understand," he asks his guide, "what's the difference between heaven and hell?"

"In heaven," answers his guide with a smile, "everyone feeds everyone else."

✦

How can you make your mealtime
"heaven" for others?

Departure

Throw out nonessential numbers. This includes
age, weight and height. Let the doctor worry about
them. That is why you pay him.

GEORGE CARLIN, STAGE COMEDIAN

WHAT NONESSENTIAL NUMBERS DO YOU CARRY
with you throughout the day? Do you constantly weigh
yourself? Do you measure your calories and count your victories
(and losses) at each meal? True, some numbers can be important –
like blood pressure, blood sugar level, etc. But some are just ways
to occupy your mind and time.

One of the keys to skillful departure from mealtime is openness and uncertainty. What would happen, for example, if you did
not weigh yourself for a day or two?

Openness does not mean you are lost, uncertain, and undecided.
It can mean that you are not stuck in the same movement, like a
machine. Uncertainty means living joyfully with not weighing yourself after a meal.

◆

Let yourself enter a period of uncertainty
and freedom after mealtime. Break a habit
and give yourself a break.

Entry

A good runner leaves no tracks.

Lao Tzu

DO YOU EVER ENTER A MEAL FEELING RELAXED and calm? Do you check your emotions at the kitchen door? When you act in this way, you wisely leave "no tracks," as Lao Tzu advises. This is not always easily accomplished, however. It requires awareness of your physical and emotional state.

Before you enter mealtime, take a moment of pause. Breathe slowly into your diaphragm. Experience your body tension. Listen to your thoughts to see if you are anxious, angry, tired, upset, and needing comfort. Accept these feelings and enter mealtime mindful of their presence.

You can release physical feelings by alternately tightening and loosening your body where you feel tension and tightness. If your shoulders are tense, for example, take a breath as you purposely tighten your muscles for up to seven seconds. Then exhale as you let the muscles relax. You can also do this for all muscle groups, including your forehead and facial muscles.

◆

Leave your physical and emotional
tracks at the kitchen door.

Choices

*I'm President of the United States, and I'm not
going to eat any more broccoli.*

GEORGE BUSH SR.

DO CERTAIN FOODS MAKE YOU REACT BY FEELING upset or angry? Do you ever feel like President Bush? After all, you are president of your own body, and you can choose to eat what you want. Understandably, the foods you were forced to eat as a child tend to lose a certain luster when you get older. It may be worthwhile, though, to become more mindful of what you might be missing.

Broccoli, for example, is part of a vegetable family rich in beta-carotene, fiber, minerals, vitamins, and more. The antioxidants it contains are also thought to be beneficial against disease. Other vegetables with these properties include cauliflower, kale, turnips, and mustard greens.

Are there certain food groups missing completely from your dietary choices? You might want to explore these gaps on your own or with a nutritionist or dietitian. Mindfulness also means knowing how to choose the nutrients that are best for you.

♦

Be mindful of which foods you routinely
ignore and learn more about them.

Preparations

*The lifework of becoming one with the
smallest daily task leads to the union of the mind
with the seasons and nature.*

SOSHITSU SEN XV, *Tea Life, Tea Mind*

WHAT IS THE SMALLEST DAILY TASK IN YOUR
kitchen preparation? Do you skip over it because it seems
unimportant or inconsequential? In truth, even the smallest task
can be highly valuable.

When I prepare food, for example, I always wash my hands first.
And if I am handling raw meat or fish, then I am mindful of washing my hands during and after the preparation so that I do not
cross-contaminate any other food or food surface.

There are no small tasks and no unimportant jobs when it comes
to cleaning your kitchen work surfaces, trays, and food. If you were
a master artist, how would you go about cleaning each utensil or
preparing to make a single cup of tea?

Remember that the place where you prepare food is as sacred
as the food itself.

✦

Experience the smallest daily kitchen task
with the greatest importance.

Rituals

Take care that your hearts are not
weighed down with overindulgence.

Luke 21:34

Is your heart ever heavy because of over-indulgence at mealtime? If so, then you might want to incorporate some kind and thoughtful words into your personal mealtime ritual blessing.

What does overindulgence mean to you? Do you define it as going off your diet plan by even a little bit? Does it mean feeling uncomfortably stuffed? Does it mean bingeing and purging? Think about your own pattern, and then think about how it makes you feel in your heart. Under the frustration and anger do you feel sadness? Do you feel a loss of hope? Do you feel overwhelmed?

Place your hand over your heart center, or clasp both hands over your heart as you say: "May my heart not be weighed down by my own expectations. May I forgive myself and know that my innermost knowing being strives for health."

Do not forget: There is still a "knowing" you – even when you overindulge.

◆

Explore expectations surrounding
overindulgence.

Eating

*If the ax is dull and its edge unsharpened, more
strength is needed but skill will bring success.*

ECCLESIASTES 10:10

WHEN "THE AX IS DULL," MINDLESS EATING RE-
SULTS. Fortunately, you can sharpen the edge of your mindfulness with skill. Sharpen your mindfulness by paying attention
to your sensations, your mind/perceptions, and your body.

Sensations are your visceral experience of the meal, including
how it tastes, looks, feels, and smells, as well as your liking or dis-
liking the food. You can practice being aware with any food.

Next, pay attention to your thoughts as you eat, including such
things as judgments and desires regarding your eating habits, diet,
and eating conflicts. Do not let anything escape the net of your
conscious awareness.

Lastly, you can cut through mindless routine by sharpening the
awareness of your body movements. This includes how you sit at
the table, pick up the fork, move the food to your mouth, how you
chew and swallow, etc. This could also include the feeling of bod-
ily fullness and hunger.

◆

Sharpen your mindfulness practices.

Community

Make the best use out of whatever
greens you have.

ZEN MASTER DOGEN, THIRTEENTH CENTURY

THE ZEN COOK DOES NOT ALWAYS HAVE HER pick of greens. Likewise, when it comes to shared or communal meals, your family, friends, and associates are the "greens" that you have to work with.

These familial and other intimate "greens" may raise certain negative emotions and feeling. For example, do you get annoyed with your family at holiday time? Do they bring what you consider to be unacceptable or unhealthy food to your meals? Do they lack etiquette and dinner conversation skills? Do they eat too much (or not enough)?

You do not get to choose all your family members. Accept the people in your life, and take responsibility for letting yourself be tolerant and mindful of how they relate to food differently than you do.

◆

How can you best accommodate
your familial "greens"?

Departure

I wish I hadn't had that final drink.

H. S. MACKINTOSH, POET

Do you ever wish you had not had that final bite – or even the next-to-the-last bite? But you did. Now you have to deal with the consequences.

What are the consequences for you? Are they physical, emotional, or spiritual? Do you try to forget it and go to sleep until the discomforting consequences go away?

First, you can deal with that last bite by accepting it and also regretting it. Regret does not mean you feel guilty or shameful. But regret is important because it demonstrates that you admit the negative consequences of your mealtime habits and that you are ready to make a change.

Secondly, forgive your less than skillful eating habits. This means you have compassion for yourself.

Thirdly, take a specific vow – such as vowing to take one less bite at your next meal. This is a small enough change that you can succeed at. Together, these three steps will help you deal with that last bite.

◆

Follow three easy steps when that
final bite hurts too much.

Entry

*When there is no firewood, fire goes out; and when
no one is quarrelsome, argument ends.*

PYTHAGORAS, GREEK MATHEMATICIAN

DO YOU POSSESS EMOTIONAL "FIREWOOD" THAT IS easily ignited at mealtime? Maybe it is so flammable that it can burst into flames at the slightest sign of distress or discomfort.

Under such situations, the best way to avoid a fire is simply this: Remove the emotional firewood before you sit down to eat. Is it your own tendency to blame yourself when your food desires overwhelm you? Is your firewood the emotions of nervousness and anxiety you feel before you quench your hunger? Is your firewood the disapproval you feel from others when they judge your eating style?

Generally, you can remove the emotions by observing them and being more mindful of them. As you recognize them, think, "There goes that feeling of being judged again," or "Here I am blaming myself." Listen and watch your emotional mealtime firewood without having to respond to it.

◆

Think how you can remove emotion
before it ignites at mealtime.

Choices

*A person who observes the rules of proper
nutrition is a person who should never be placed
in charge of a barbecue.*

DAVE BARRY, SYNDICATED HUMORIST

HOW DO YOU MINDFULLY APPROACH FOOD CHOICES when invited to a party? Do summer barbecues, for example, present a challenge for you? Grilled burgers, hot dogs, baked potatoes, coleslaw, and potato salad are perfect for some. For others, this is everything they want to avoid.

When invited to barbecues, I usually select from the food that I feel is best for me under the circumstances. However, you may want to go further. After all, you need to take responsibility for what you eat.

Ask if you can bring some of your own food to cook on the grill. This could be almost anything, from fish to soy burgers to vegetables. Do not be shy about telling the host of your food preferences. From my own experience, I have cooked just about anything on the grill – from whole turkeys and salmon to kabobs and apple pies. If you are mindful, you can take part in summer food festivities.

◆

Let your choices be known at summer meals.

Preparations

The Master does his job and then stops.
He understands that the universe is
forever out of control.

LAO TZU

WHEN PREPARING YOUR MEAL, DO YOU KNOW when to stop? Are you a perfectionist? Do you have to cook every meal (or your meal) because no one else can do it right? Do you exhaust yourself by preparing food for hours, then complain that you get no help?

All of these are possible signals that you may be holding on too tightly. Maybe it is your way of making sure you are appreciated or managing some emotional distaste or resistance. At some point, you can relinquish control over preparation. You can either let go a little on your own or let someone else stir the soup for a while. The other alternative is burnout. So, how do you let go?

You can think about it all you want, but that does not get it done. You can only let go by letting go.

◆

When you hold too tightly,
let go a little today.

Rituals

The ritual is One
The food is One
We who offer the food are One
The fire of hunger is also One
All action is One
We who understand this are One.

HINDU BLESSING

 DO YOU EVER FEEL LIKE YOU ARE OF TWO MINDS at mealtime? There is the "good" you who sticks to your eating plan and the "bad" you who eats every temptation in sight.

The Hindu ritual blessing, above, can help you to experience all of your mealtime actions and thoughts – even if they contradict one another – as all stemming from the same knowing source. This knowing transcends your dualistic, or relativistic, thought patterns and conflicts.

It may appear illogical that two completely different thoughts can be united. But is it not true that your one mind creates all the opposing thoughts you have about food? And when you think about it, the idea of you being either over- or underweight would have no meaning without the opposite dynamic.

◆

If nondual thinking makes sense to you, add
this to your mealtime ritual blessing.

Eating

*In general, mankind, since the improvement of
cookery, eats twice as much as nature requires.*

BENJAMIN FRANKLIN

DO YOU FEEL THAT YOU EAT MORE THAN YOU NEED?
Obviously, eating more than you require is not new. However, people were probably more physically active one or two hundred years ago than they are today.

There are two good tools for when you may eat too much. The first is slowing down your eating, and the second is using mindfulness to watch and guard against eating too much. (Exercise is a good practice, but not if its sole purpose is to burn off calories from overeating. Exercise for the sake of health.)

One good way to slow eating and aid digestion is to chew your food up to twenty-five times for each bite before swallowing. (Some people practice one hundred chews per bite.)

Also, use mindfulness to set an intention before every movement you make at mealtime such as mentally saying, "I intend to lift the fork," "I intend to raise the spoon to my mouth," etc.

◆

Moderate your quantity of food at
today's meal by slowing down and
using mindful intention.

Community

I come from a home where gravy is a beverage.

ERMA BOMBECK, SYNDICATED COLUMNIST

DOES YOUR FAMILY POSSESS SOME EATING STYLES and foods that you absolutely adore? Are there other family habits, however, that make you want to cringe and hide your head under the napkin? Either way, you are not alone.

You cannot get much more personal than eating. Children often view their family's eating patterns as normal – even if those patterns are disordered. There are families, for example, where children are encouraged to eat excessive amounts of dessert at meals – even when the children do not want them. The point here is not to get judgmental, but to be compassionate.

Compassion and mindful self-awareness can help you find your own way to health when you come from a home where "gravy is a beverage."

✦

What old family eating pattern do you love
or hate? How can you find your own way?

Departure

Fasting is the best medicine.

INDIAN PROVERB

A COMPLETE MEAL IS ONE THAT LEAVES YOU bliss-fulfilled and wanting no more (or less). With this kind of deep experience, you can depart mealtime without the need or desire to nibble mindlessly until your next meal. If your recent meal is truly bliss-fulfilled, then you can naturally balance it with follow-up fasting and digesting (a good "medicine").

But when a meal leaves you unsatisfied, then you need to explore why. Is your remaining hunger physical or emotional? Do you really eat enough food? Is there enough variety to satisfy your body's nutritional needs? Is there emotional turmoil in your life at this time?

There is no magic pill to help you find peace with the meal you have just eaten. Remember, you can always use the entire process of eating – entry, preparation, food choices, ritual, eating, and community – to help you find your way back to fulfillment.

◆

Let your bliss-fulfilling meal cultivate natural
fasting until your next meal.

Entry

*Each step taken in mindfulness can be
a step taken in gratitude for your entire body and
state of well-being.*

DONALD ALTMAN, *Living Kindness*

DOES YOUR BODY LEAD YOU TO A MEALTIME (OR snack) by walking quickly or being tense? Your body's tension and posture prior to eating can mask emotional blockages. You can naturally balance and release this emotion by engaging your body's mindfulness.

Begin by placing your attention on your body. Do you feel stress in your shoulders, neck, arms, chest, legs, or stomach? Once you identify the tense area – for example, your shoulders – inhale for a count of three as you consciously tighten those muscles. Then relax that muscle group as you exhale, letting the tension and stress go.

Next be mindful of your posture. Is your body slouching, upright, rigid, flexible, energized, or fatigued? How does your posture reflect your feelings about the upcoming meal? Stand in place for a moment and readjust your posture until you feel balanced and grounded. Let your stance reflect a feeling of well-being, free of fear and doubt. As you enter your kitchen or eating place, carry mindfulness and peace forward into your mealtime.

◆

Let mindfulness of your body set the rhythm
for your upcoming meal.

Choices

Everything you see I owe to spaghetti.

SOPHIA LOREN

 DO YOU DEMONIZE CERTAIN FOODS EVEN AS YOU eat them – or as someone else does? As Sophia Loren affirms, carbohydrates are not necessarily evil.

For this meditation, you will closely experience your feelings and thoughts around tempting, or what you consider "bad," foods. Realize that this will not make you lose control. Instead, it will eventually give you greater freedom of choice because you will lessen your conflict over food.

Try this: Examine your desires in detail as you restrain from eating a tempting food. What is the source of your craving for it? Do you desire the taste or feeling of comfort the food will offer you? If you stay with your thoughts, feelings, and desires long enough, you may notice that they change or fade away – even for a moment. Even if you decide to eat the food, continue to watch your feelings as they rise into being and eventually dissolve.

◆

Explore how thoughts and feelings of
"bad" foods do not last forever by watching
them rise and fall.

Preparations

[Cooking] tasks and rhythms remain, for me,
something both holy and fun.

CRESCENT DRAGONWAGON, COOKBOOK AUTHOR

 HAVE YOU EVER DONE SOMETHING IN THE KITCHEN that was both holy and fun? Even the most mundane tasks can be done with a sense of sacredness and fun.

I distinctly remember the time, for example, that I visited Brother Roy at Mount Calvary Monastery in Santa Barbara, California. My purpose was to interview him about his wonderful, multigrain monastery-made bread and his approach to food. I met Brother Roy in the kitchen where he was washing dishes, pots, and utensils. I asked if I could help, and together we stood washing and drying the dishes.

We worked in silence, letting the cleaning be a kind of sacred and holy communication between us – a way of acknowledging that nothing more need be said or felt.

Be silent as you prepare and clean up your meal. Let the work fill up the silence with wholeness – and whole-liness.

◆

Experience the whole-liness of
preparation in sublime silence.

Rituals

Are there graces for lettuce, Lord? . . .
For I need help in becoming the healthier person I
want to be. Hold up for me a mirror of the new
creation you see me to be, for I need a companion
at this table, Lord.

MARGARET ANNE HUFFMAN, *Grace for Dieting*

 DO YOU EVER FIND IT DIFFICULT TO BE GRATEFUL
for the food on your plate when you are dieting? Are you
ever unhappy or resentful about having to eat a restricted diet
(whether it is your choice or health-related)? The ritual blessing
above may help deal with your feelings.

Even if you are eating healthfully, you may be suffering emotionally because of your transition to a new way of living with food.
A ritual blessing can offer compassion and hope.

Ask for help from the divine so that you can make peace with the
part of you that wants to hold onto old – though unhealthy – habits.
You may also want to add:"May I have compassion for all of me, the
me that is changing and the me that does not want to change, as I
undertake this new path to healthy eating."

♦

Say a grace for your diet or new,
healthy eating.

Eating

Preach not to others what they should eat,
but eat as becomes you and be silent.

EPICTETUS, GREEK PHILOSOPHER

HAVE YOU EVER INTENTIONALLY EATEN A MEAL in which you avoided being critical of yourself or others? This is an expression of kindness and silence by what is not said. Being kind is about more than not speaking – it is also about what you say and how you say it while at the dinner table.

When you place your focus on being considerate of others at mealtime, you extend your mindfulness beyond your own experience of eating. As I learned in the monastery, for example, the monks always place some focus on others around them – all the while speaking only as much as required. The result is that no one is criticized for eating too much or not enough. It is assumed that each person knows what is best for him at that particular moment.

◆

Experience the silence that spreads wisdom
and acceptance – of self and others.

Community

*I vow to offer joy to one person in the
morning and to help to relieve the grief of one
person in the afternoon.*

THICH NHAT HANH

DO YOU USE YOUR MEALTIME AS A CONDUIT TO generate joy and bliss? All it takes to raise your meal from the mundane to the sacred is to use it as a tool for living kindness.

Mealtime is ideal for spreading love and generosity. First, it is a naturally communal activity. Secondly, eating is a nourishing act of survival and caring for oneself. Thirdly, food is a common touchstone that brings all beings together – since all need to eat and are dependent on the earth for food.

Each day, become aware of these three principles for finding communal joy and bliss in food. Then, share these blessings with others. For example, share an uplifting story with someone at mealtime, offer food to someone in need, and take a mealtime vow to help one person today.

◆

Use your mealtime to spread bliss and joy.

Departure

Whenever I feel like exercise I lie down
until the feeling passes.

ROBERT MAYNARD HUTCHINS,
AMERICAN EDUCATOR

HOW ACTIVE ARE YOU AFTER A MEAL? DO YOU usually sleep after a meal? Or, if you are unhappy with what you eat, do you feel compelled to go out and exercise off the calories? Any of these behaviors might mean that you need more balance after mealtime.

Depending on what you eat, drowsiness may not be unusual. But if you are always sluggish after eating, then your diet might need adjustment. Be sure that you balance after-meal resting with an activity such as exercise or walking.

Likewise, if all you do is exercise after mealtime, then you need to find moderation. Linking eating with either excessive rest or exercise can be a recipe for unhealthy and perhaps compulsive behavior.

◆

Find balance and bliss after mealtime
by feeling into your natural rhythm
for rest and exercise.

Entry

Small doubt, small enlightenment;
big doubt, big enlightenment.

KOREAN ZEN MASTER NINE MOUNTAINS

DO YOU EVER ENTER A MEAL DOUBTING YOUR DIET? Do you doubt if there is a healthy balance between your exercise and your eating? Doubt is one of the obstacles to effort. With doubt, you can shut down or just stop trying.

The good news is that you can easily transform doubt from a weakness and into a strength by having the wisdom to seek more truth and information. One famous doubter was Saint Thomas, from whom the term "Doubting Thomas" originated. But like Saint Thomas, it is important for you to doubt and question. Through this process you can refine and gain faith in your dietary choices.

Here are some ways to work with doubt: Do more reading on the subject. Pay attention to the effect of foods and choices on your body energy and digestion. Get the opinion of a nutritionist, doctor, dietitian, or other health professional that you trust.

◆

Use the wisdom of doubting to gain more
information and faith about your eating.

Choices

*We load up on the bran in the morning so we'll
live forever. Then we spend the rest of the day
living like there's no tomorrow.*

LEE IACOCCA, U.S. BUSINESSMAN

DO YOU LOAD UP ON THE BRAN IN THE MORNING,
or at lunch, only to lose control of your food choices later
on? When you do this, what is really going on?

There are several reasons why you might make skillful food
choices for part of the day and then lose focus at other times. It
may be that you have more control over your choices at some meals
than others. Restaurants, for example, might not have the options
you prefer.

Another reason could be that you are not really in touch with
your body and the stress levels around you. I know one person, for
example, who struggles with overeating only at work, but not else-
where. This individual denies work stress even though all the signs
of it are present.

How are your choices acting as medication, such as medicating
your unhappiness at home or your stress at work?

◆

Discover when you eat "right" and when you
disappoint yourself. Then, look for the truth.

Preparations

Art is food for the soul.

DARLENE JONES, *Cooking with Spirit*

FINDING BLISS WITH FOOD CAN COME IN THE smallest of details as you prepare your meal. When you make food an art, as many chefs do, you begin to appreciate it in ways you never thought possible.

For example, have you ever heard of a zester? It is a hand-held utensil that takes off the outermost, oil-scented part of a lemon rind for cooking – without going to the bitter inner portion. The point here is not to fill your kitchen with innumerable products that you will rarely use. The idea is to put more "zest" and art in your preparation by exploring something new – whether it happens to be a utensil, ingredient, presentation, or recipe.

Look around your kitchen with a set of fresh eyes. Appreciate with gratitude the tools that daily make your life easier, and the plates and dishes that add color and art to your soul food.

◆

Give thanks for the artful expression of
preparation in today's meal.

Rituals

These are the true drops of love. . . .
Be faithful in small things because it is in
them that your strength lies.

MOTHER TERESA,
The True Drops of Love or, How Does a Lamp Burn

DO YOU SEEK THE ONE PERFECT RITUAL BLESSING that would diminish your food struggles and offer peace at mealtime? You are not alone. The truth, however, may be closer to the idea expressed in this poem written by Mother Teresa.

Instead of looking for that one great truth about food, use Mother Teresa's words as a ritual blessing to help ground you in the truth and strength of small things.

What are the small things this blessing talks about? Well, think for a moment that it takes many drops of water to fill your glass. It takes many bites to make a full meal. It takes many moments of mindful awareness to bring fulfillment. Do not be lured into dissatisfaction because a step is small and does not seem to make a difference. It does.

◆

Let this ritual blessing support your strength
in "small things" that you do.

Eating

*Food eaten at a table is better for you than
food eaten hunched over a desk, at a counter, or
driving in a car. And I believe that, wherever
you do it, hurried eating has ruined more digestive
systems than foie gras.*

PETER MAYLE, *Encore Provence*

 DO YOU EAT WHILE ON THE RUN? WHILE DRIVING to work? While working – either at the office or at home? Do not feel bad about this. The pace of American life has been catered to by the ease of fast-food restaurants. Perhaps that is why Americans nibble and eat at all times of the day. There is eating – which can conveniently be done anytime – and then there is savoring a meal. A meal lets you eat with your focus on the food, lets you trade your pace for a moment of peace.

If less than half of your eating is a "meal," then eating quickly is probably an ingrained, habitual part of your life.

Fortunately, you can still eat fast food mindfully. You can still chew twenty-five times and slow down and taste the food. You can still take a mindful breath and pause before ordering. You can still decide to eat a meal.

◆

Become aware of how often
you have a meal.

Community

*Everyone needs beauty as well as bread, places to
play in and pray in where Nature may heal and
cheer and give strength to body and soul alike.*

JOHN MUIR, NATURALIST AND WRITER

DO YOU EVER COMBINE FOOD WITH NATURE?
Do you ever eat outside or bring the joy of nature indoors
as you dine? As the great naturalist John Muir eloquently describes,
bread, beauty, and nature are inseparable "to body and soul alike."

Communing with nature is another way to experience community while eating. You can do this in many ways. Just the other
day, for example, my wife and I drove to a nearby farm to pick tomatoes, cucumbers, and yellow peppers off the vine. Walking between
the long rows of vegetables, with open fields on all sides, was exhilarating. At that moment I was in communion with the farmers,
the soil, the plants, the earth, and the other pickers who had come
to gather food.

✦

Find a way to bring the joy of nature and
your meal in communion with one another.

Departure

*Without an efficient system of waste
removal we would rapidly poison ourselves;
moreover, as any gardener or farmer knows, the
products of elimination nourish the earth.*

PHILIP ZALESKI AND PAUL KAUFMAN, *Gifts of the Spirit*

EACH TIME YOU EAT FOOD, AS WELL AS ELIMINATE food waste from your body, you witness the miraculous workings of a biological system developed over thousands of years. Your body absorbs food's energy to create new cells and regenerate the body. It eliminates the rest.

This process is extremely complex, but your body manages it with amazing efficiency. Yet, this part of your body's operation is often ignored or not openly talked about. Elimination is a signal of how well your body is working. Regular or irregular bowel movements can tell a lot about your inner health and well-being. So, too, can intestinal problems such as irritable bowel syndrome and colitis. I have one friend, for example, who takes two capsules of liquid garlic after dinner to promote elimination and a healthy colon.

Take some time after meal to reflect on your body's elimination process. Be thankful for it as part of your sacred process of being.

◆

Appreciate with joy how your body absorbs
and eliminates what it needs for well-being.

Entry

If you reject the food, ignore the customs,
fear the religion and avoid the people,
you might better stay home.

JAMES MICHENER

WHEN YOU ENTER MEALTIME, DO EMOTIONS such as fear, anxiety, anger, and sadness make it difficult for you to digest the entire experience? How you accept or reject a food experience depends on how you feel as you enter mealtime.

For many, disappointment around food stems from setting unreasonable expectations before you even sit down to eat. Taking one bite too many or eating the wrong food taints your whole meal. If you measure your mealtime success by such rigid guidelines, then you may be setting yourself up for failure.

Mindfulness lets you eat (and live) without expectation and being a slave to your emotions. You can do this by letting go of your food expectations. Let mindful chewing and breathing slow you down as you trust in your personal wisdom of how much and what to eat.

✦

Let go of your mealtime expectations and
trust in your food wisdom.

Choices

Our deepest self-knowledge resides in the body,
which a great deal of the time does not speak the
same language as the mind.

ANNEMARIE COLBIN, *Food and Healing*

DOES YOUR MIND SHARE THE SAME LANGUAGE as your body when it comes to choosing your meal? When your mind wants to eat one thing and your body wants another, you may feel upset about your dietary choices and feel the difference in your body. How can the mental and physical aspects of your being find mutual peace?

One approach that can harmonize your mind and body is heightened awareness of each moment that you make a food choice. When you think about it, selecting your food takes only a split second of your time. Yet you spend many more moments eating that choice!

As you look at the menu, grocery shelf, or food in your cupboard, listen to your mind's emotional reactions. What is each moment-to-moment thought you have as you consider each food?

By waiting an extra moment, you give yourself a second longer to let yourself feel to what your body needs.

✦

Spend a moment more listening
to your thoughts and cravings before
choosing for today's meal.

Preparations

We stand at a fork in the road.

POPULAR SAYING

HAVE YOU EVER TAKEN A STAND ON FOOD? By that, I mean that sometimes you need to make a stand with your fork and spoon – by limiting what you let into your mouth.

How familiar are you with the ingredients in your favorite cereals, candies, dairy products, packaged foods, and sodas, etc.? Many contain a variety of food coloring, additives, and preservatives.

According to the ancient food laws of Judaism and Islam, for example, certain foods are recommended while others are prohibited. But consider many modern foods and additives that did not exist hundreds of years ago? Islam's elegant answer is this: Each of us needs to take personal responsibility for learning if a food is *mashbooh*, or suspect.

Personally, I used to drink a lot of diet sodas until information I learned about artificial sweeteners tilted these into my personal suspect category for me. The Internet and books can help you learn more about your own "suspect" foods.

◆

What foods in your diet are "suspect"?

Rituals

Nothing is imperfect. The pebble equals the ruby.
A frog is as beautiful as any seraphim.

ANGELUS SILESIUS,
SEVENTEENTH-CENTURY GERMAN MYSTIC

DO YOU GET EASILY UPSET WHEN YOU MAKE A mistake with your perfect diet plan? You may discover that trying to be perfect equates into becoming tense and anxious when it comes to eating. A ritual blessing that contains the essence of the one above can let you accept the regular, daily perfection that is present in every meal, whether you follow your dietary guidelines or do not.

Acknowledging your regular perfection is another way of saying that you accept yourself for who you are – whatever your choices may be. With regular perfection, you can experience peace with your meal instead of struggle. Regular perfection does not mean you stop trying. You can always continue to apply your effort and discipline. But you can do so with more joy and acceptance and equanimity.

◆

May you accept your every meal and bite as
perfect for where you are at this moment.

Eating

The truth is that good and bad coexist;
sour and sweet coexist. They aren't really
opposed to each other.

PEMA CHÖDRÖN, *Start Where You Are*

ARE YOU EVER AT WAR WITH YOUR DINNER? Do you fight over what and how much of a particular food to eat? Do you deny, weigh, portion, and nibble at your food? When you experience this inner battle over food opposites, then savoring food and experiencing it fully is difficult because there is always the idea that something is missing.

This is the reason why most diets do not work: When you deny yourself that pie, ice cream, or chips, then you create an opposite and equal (or greater) desire for what is being denied! This is simple cause and effect.

But what if you slowly practiced healthy moderation in place of denial? This lets you slowly change a habit, by taking one less bite of offending food – and one more bite of desirable food – than you did the meal before.

✦

Be aware of your inner food struggle and
try moderation at today's meal.

Community

Fasting is like a solitary walk under the stars.
We alone must take that first step.

DONALD ALTMAN, *Art of the Inner Meal*

HAVE YOU EVER TRIED FASTING FOR ANY PERIOD of time? Fasting is a very personal experience. It is also a communal encounter that unites people in their quest for spiritual energy and focus. Most biblical fasts, for example, are twenty-four hours long. Some, like Islam's Ramadan fast, begins at sunrise and ends at sunset for an entire month. Ramadan's group fast does more than unite people around dedication to God. Shared meals after sunset reveal the importance of sharing and the sweet blessing of life that is provided by food.

If you have never fasted, consider a short, moderate, and compassionate fast – one where you can fast for only as long as you feel is safe and comfortable. Adapt this fast to your body, for example, by allowing yourself to drink liquids or other foods during your fast period.

Even a short fast offers many benefits: It can help you appreciate food, give your body a rest, increase concentration, and give you freedom from your food desires and emotions. (Talk to your doctor or health professional before undergoing any kind of fast.)

◆

Reflect on how to undertake a
compassionate and moderate fast as part of
a religious tradition or by yourself.

Departure

I believe in the pears and apples of autumn,
the pumpkins, the blue-gray squashes that
nourish our bodies with their meat, our spirits
with their beauty.

THELMA J. PALMER, POET

THIS DATE HAPPENS TO MARK THE AUTUMNAL equinox, a time for harvesting and gathering the fruits of spring's labor. Likewise, the transition of the seasons is a good time for you to take stock of your mealtime progress to date.

What new seeds and mindful attitudes did you cultivate throughout the summer season? Do you find more self-acceptance of your eating struggles and conflicts? As you depart today's meal, can you recognize a change in your awareness of food? Where is your food journey leading as you enter the new season?

As you depart today's meal, also reflect on your gratitude for the food of the earth and your ancestors – two other important aspects of traditional harvest festivals. Let yourself revel in joy and bliss of your achievement and deeper understanding of the role of food in your life.

◆

Take heart in your own harvest of knowing
and mindfulness in the season of your life.

Entry

I believe a leaf of grass is no less than the
journey-work of the stars.

WALT WHITMAN

THINK BACK FOR A MOMENT ON YOUR LAST MEAL. Did anything surprise you? Did the foods make an impact in terms of nutrition, flavor, and deeper meaning? When meals are mundane and ordinary, then you may be missing out on the ever-present miracle that food represents – just like Whitman's "leaf of grass."

As you enter your next journey with food, you can shift into sacred space just by taking a mindful walk. In this way, you allow the precious moment of your upcoming to unfold before you without expectations.

Walk mindfully by (1) setting an intention to step forward, (2) following up with action, and (3) observing all your movements in detail. If your thoughts stray, simply return to the intention to take a step. Then, experience your meal with intention, action, and observation in the moment.

◆

Awaken to each fresh moment
of food's sacredness.

Choices

We are what we think....
Speak or act with an impure mind
And trouble will follow you
As the wheel follows the ox that draws the cart.

BUDDHA, *Dhammapada*

IS YOUR DESIRE FOR A CERTAIN FOOD NOT SATIS-fied until you eat it? How strongly do your desires dictate food choices? You can better understand your food choices by rating the impulses and desires that drive them "as the ox that draws the cart."

On a scale of 1 to 10, rate how frequently you choose food because of very strong and persistent thoughts and emotions. If almost all the time you choose food because of a thought or emotion, score a 10. If about half of the time you choose food because of strong thoughts or emotions, score a 5. If you rarely choose food because of emotion or desire, but because you sense they are best for your body, mind, and spirit, you can score a 1.

Take note of those periods when you rate higher on the food desire scale. Are you more stressed, for example, when you score a 10 than a 5?

✦

Explore how often your food
choices are driven by your desires,
thoughts, and emotions.

Preparations

*What saves man is to take a step. Then
another step. It is always the same step,
but you have to take it.*

ANTOINE DE SAINT-EXUPÉRY, PILOT AND POET

DO YOU PREPARE YOUR MEAL WITH COURAGE? Or do you pause at some point and think it would be easier to eat out? What stops you from creating meals or using new ingredients? Do the same emotions that hold you back from enjoying a meal also create an obstacle to your preparing it?

Fear, for example, can block many things, even preparing french toast. Suppose you have never made french toast. You may fear that you will not prepare it as perfectly as your favorite restaurant. Or you may fear the ingredients will be so tempting that you will eat more than you should. You end up conflicted over the french toast that you want but fight against internally.

Is there a middle ground to preparation? Can you, for example, make a single slice of french toast? Can you prepare other healthy items in an attractive way that that will supplement your french toast?

◆

Explore fear of preparation and
find the middle ground.

Rituals

*This farewell comes from a forgiving leaf
that skipped with the others and then found
a lucky storm that brought me here. Listen –
hold on as long as you can, then thrust forth:
make truth your home.*

WILLIAM STAFFORD, POET

 DO YOU TRUST IN YOUR FOOD WISDOM? WHAT have you learned in your many seasons of gaining sustenance and caring for you body that you can use now? The sentiments in the poem by William Stafford ask us to trust in what really matters as we grow older with wisdom and experience.

Your inner, knowing voice knows the difference between wellness and sickness. The fact that you may struggle with food means that you are in the process of finding balance and maturity. This process is natural, just as all of nature goes through stages from infancy to adulthood to maturity.

Incorporate a wise ritual blessing like the one above when you need strength to listen to your wise, mature inner voice. Have faith.

It is there if you will listen.

◆

Listen and trust in your many
seasons of food wisdom.

Eating

Mr. Duffy lived a short distance from his body.

JAMES JOYCE, *Ulysses*

HOW FAR DO YOU LIVE FROM YOUR BODY WHILE you eat? Do you feel comfortable with your body's shape and size? Or do you feel like you inhabit a body that does not co-operate with you?

Feeling at home in your body is necessary to feel your real physical hunger and to accept your body's weight, shape, and size. If you struggle with food, you may live a distance from your body.

One way you can find out is to time yourself as you mindfully focus on eating something for a full five minutes. Take a single raisin (slice of orange, peanut, etc.) and experience it totally using all your senses. The higher your comfort level, the more ease you may feel with your body. If you become tense, simply stop and feel the discomfort. Be more aware of the thoughts and feelings that are present.

✦

Experience comfort or discomfort
with your body as you eat.

Community

After a good dinner, one can forgive anybody,
even one's relations.

OSCAR WILDE, IRISH DRAMATIST AND NOVELIST

DO YOU FEEL CALMER AND MORE FORGIVING OF others during a meal? Or do you feel anxious or argumentative? If forgiveness – toward yourself or others – is important to you, than a community meal offers you an opportunity for experiencing and practicing it.

Although forgiveness is not always asked for at mealtime, it is ever present. Because each time you eat, you receive and absorb the gift of life from another living thing. If you can forgive yourself for this, then you can certainly forgive another for pushing your buttons at mealtime or during the day.

You do not have to let mealtime become a contest where there are winners and losers. Focus on the wonder of your food and the sacredness of those who are with you at this moment.

◆

Experience forgiveness toward
others by focusing on the sacredness
of food and community.

Departure

Without silence, there is no ecstasy.

KATHLEEN NORRIS, *Amazing Grace*

DO YOU EVER EXPERIENCE A SENSE OF BLISS AND joy after your meal? How you approach the moments after your meal can make all the difference.

While silence enhances mindfulness during mealtime, you can use it to experience the bliss that follows your meal. First, be aware of your present routine. Do you quickly clean up your meal so you can get on with more "pleasant" activities? Do you go right back to work because your lunch period is short?

Personally, whenever I have a short lunch, I often try to take a minute in silence before returning to work.

In one minute you can feel the bliss of food's energy and the miracle of your body's digestive process. You can feel all the blessings that come from having food on your plate and in your stomach.

◆

Take even one minute in silence after eating
to feel the bliss and blessings of your meal.

Entry

May you be inscribed for life in the New Year.

TRADITIONAL JEWISH NEW YEAR GREETING

AS A NEW SEASON AND THE NEW YEAR APPROACH, you can "inscribe," or make a difference for yourself in life, through the celebration of food. Food, after all, supports your life. Why not enjoy it?

For this day, explore food. Let yourself enter mealtime with a sense of wonderment and openness. Try a restaurant or meal that is new for you. Decide beforehand that you will eat moderately and let your body guide you toward what and how much to eat.

Also, celebrate by letting go of your expectations and emotions about the new meal. You do not have to feel guilty for breaking dietary rules – or good for keeping them – but simply skillful or unskillful.

◆

May you inscribe your coming year with
a new approach to food.

Choices

Let food be your medicine and
medicine be your food.

HIPPOCRATES

IS FOOD REALLY MEDICINE? THINK FOR A MOMENT about the purpose and properties of food. The purpose of food is to give you strength, well being, and energy. But there are all kinds of foods. The wrong foods can harm your body and put it at risk; the proper ones can heal, as well as guard you from aging and illness.

Do you remember a time when your doctor or other health professional recommended a dietary change? What did you do? Some just find another doctor – which only works in the short-term. Eventually, the consequences of your food choices will catch up with you. Your body is not a mechanical device, but an integrated organic miracle that is perfectly tuned to work with the natural environment.

Become more aware of your body's reaction to the foods that offer natural medicine and health.

◆

What benefit do you get from "natural"
food? Add one or more of these medicine
foods to today's diet.

Preparations

What's the use of watching?
A watched pot never boils.

E. S. GASKELL

MEAL PREPARATION AND COOKING REQUIRE MUL-
tiple skills. But unless you carefully watch what you are
doing, you may run into difficulties – such as pots boiling over,
sinks running over, microwaves scorching food, and patience growing thin.

Fortunately, you can eliminate mindless preparation accidents
and mistakes wherever you prepare your meal – in the kitchen or
vending machine area. You can simply activate mindfulness with
the following intention: "May I use the power of focused attention
to witness each step of preparation. May I see and experience each
moment fresh and for the first time, without distraction."

Now, closely examine every detail of your preparation. Notice the
movement of your body. Watch as you set the temperature on a
stovetop or microwave. Be present the entire time. And when you
are not, be mindful of that, too!

◆

Do what you can to remove distractions
and watch your entire preparation
with total awareness.

Rituals

O Earth, wrap me in your leaves – heal me. . . .
Let my wounds become fertile gardens
and . . . let me live again.

ALLA RENÉE BOZARTH, EPISCOPAL PRIEST

ARE YOU TIRED AND EXHAUSTED OF THINKING about your food and weight issues? Do you ever just wish you could make it all go away? Well, there is no magic pill to make emotional eating habits disappear. But you can heal and promote wellness by applying effort in this moment!

If there is a secret to healing, it is that you have the power to recognize how negative emotions and thoughts around food have consequences. You can recall and substitute positive thoughts with a healing ritual blessing like the one above. Acknowledge your wounds, but focus on your strength and courage. As part of your blessing, you can also visualize a time when you chose food wisely.

Practice your visualization as follows: Focus on a positive eating experience – one where you felt satisfied, skillful, and good about what and how much you ate. Specifically recall the room, people, smells, tastes, and your emotional state as you ate that meal. Recall and use this positive memory in challenging times.

◆

Remember your strengths and call
upon them during your mealtime blessing
to help you right now.

Eating

*In eating, a third of the stomach should be filled with
food, a third with drink, and the rest left empty.*

THE TALMUD

DO YOU ROUTINELY EAT ALL THE FOOD ON YOUR
plate and leave your meal feeling stuffed? Do food cravings
overwhelm you? Do you know that you are eating too much but
feel distraught and unable to stop yourself? If so, you may fit the pro-
file of chronic overeating.

You need mindfulness to (1) slow down your eating, (2) listen
to your cravings, and (3) listen to your body.

First, slow your eating by becoming aware of your breath. Take
a breath between bites. Chew (up to twenty-five times) before
swallowing.

Next, listen to your thoughts, including the emotional hunger,
neediness, and appetite that drive you. Do not condemn your emotions and cravings; at the same time, know that you have another
inner voice that seeks moderation and wellness. Both can exist side
by side even as you slow down your eating.

Finally, feel your body, stomach, and digestion. Feel when you
have had enough food, even though your mind craves more.

◆

Practice leaving some food on your plate and
some space in your stomach at today's meal. (If you
do not like to waste food, give yourself permission
to stop eating anyway.)

Community

*My wife broke our dog of eating at the table –
she let him taste it.*

PAT COOPER, COMEDIAN

DO YOU EVER GO TO A POTLUCK ONLY TO FIND that eating spirals out of control and you taste a little of everything? Or do you get upset because the food is not what you consider healthy or appropriate?

If you struggle with food and diet, potluck dinners can be good practice for learning how to discriminate between the food you desire and the food your body really requires. It can also help you witness your limiting and judgmental views of yourself and others.

Is the food you bring to the potluck consistent with your typical dietary choices? Or do you reward yourself by bringing treats and make this meal an exception?

At such times, it is useful to state an intention beforehand: "I intend to stay mindful of what food my body really needs. And though I may be tempted, I will be mindful of my desires and emotions, too."

◆

State your intention before any mealtime
gathering to stay mindful.

Departure

*More people will die from hit-or-miss eating
than from hit-and-run driving.*

DUNCAN HINES, *Adventures in Good Eating*

 DO YOU EVER EMOTIONALLY BEAT YOURSELF UP after eating? Do you blame yourself for eating too much (or not enough)? It is okay to think about your last meal, but do you really gain anything by berating yourself afterward?

Take alternative action to (1) stop the emotional browbeating, (2) live with the immediate consequences, such as poor digestion, feeling uncomfortably full, etc., and (3) take a vow to be mindful and plan better at your next meal.

First, listen to your emotions, knowing that all the one-sided thoughts, guilt, and shame you may feel are slanted. There are always two perspectives. Take a moment to think of a more balanced view, such as sometimes you eat a little less, pick a healthy food, do not obsess about food, etc.

Next, accept that how you feel physically is a consequence of your earlier thoughts and actions – which you have the ability to change. Lastly, explore how to eat a mindful, beneficial meal the next time. Even just one less (more) bite is a more skillful action!

◆

Take a vow to be mindful in planning
your next meal. Use mindfulness tools daily
and it gets easier.

Entry

May suffering ones be suffering free,
May the fear struck fearless be,
May grieving ones shed all grief,
May all beings find relief.

BUDDHIST BLESSING

DO YOU FIND THAT YOU HAVE A LOT OF NEGATIVE chatter in your mind before you eat? Unhealthy emotions can be an obstacle to effort. They can even cause you to use food as medication – which is not a long-term answer to feeling better.

When emotions derail your best intentions, you can (1) write down your thoughts and emotions, (2) focus on your mindful breath or walking, and (3) focus on your strengths.

First, writing down emotional thoughts – such as, "I feel bad, gross, disgusting, etc." – can give you some separation from demanding and critical thoughts. And it shifts you from the subjective to the objective realm where you can better engage your mind-body-spirit to get unstuck.

Next, focus on your breath or walking for at least five minutes. This builds up your attention, positive energy, and calmness. Finally, focus on your strengths. Decide upon one small action – such as taking one less (or more) bite of food for your health and well-being.

◆

Overcome unhealthy emotions
before your next meal.

Choices

All I ask of food is that it doesn't harm me.

MICHAEL PALIN, WRITER AND COMEDIAN

DO FOOD CHOICES HARM YOU IN SOME WAY? Do they make you feel angry, disappointed, frustrated, or upset? Do they leave you bloated, sick, or feeling helpless? If so, then you already know that your choices, or actions, have an effect on your mind and body.

The next step is to make more skillful choices. But first, you need to accept that your present choices carry a lifetime of energy and habit behind them. Thus, your emotional and physical reactions have a lifetime of energy behind them as well! Where to begin?

Start by knowing your current choices can be changed over time by applying industrial strength awareness. I say "industrial strength" because just knowing your choices is not enough. Even an unskillful choice may offer you something – such as emotional comfort, attention from others, temporary relief, numbness, etc. – that makes it a habit. Learn what that is.

◆

Explore what you get from an unskillful habit.

Preparations

Sometimes it is the only worthwhile product you can salvage from a day: what you make to eat. . . .
Cooking therefore, can keep a person who tries sane.

JOHN IRVING, AUTHOR

DO YOU OFTEN HAVE DAYS WHEN YOU HARDLY have time to catch a meal? Do you find your life speeding up so fast that you are totally tense – especially when it comes to enjoying your evening meal? If so, then you will be glad to know that cooking and preparation are great ways to center both yourself and your emotions.

Cooking grounds you to the earth. It brings you back to the basics and back to what is elemental and vital: to eat and sustain and nourish yourself. (When you think about it, this is where all of your activities are directed.) By cooking you care for yourself (and perhaps others), and you return to what really matters.

Understandably, you may be tempted to settle for the fast-food solution. If you do this, you can still be mindful, but it may not settle you down and offer deep satisfaction because preparation is so involving. (Also, if your time is limited or you are really exhausted, you could try to make food beforehand.)

◆

Let cooking center your emotions as you
nourish and take care of yourself.

Rituals

Two sisters by the door, a pair
Their harmony is something rare
A love of cooking both do share
But it's platonic, their cupboard is bare
The food they had brought no longer there.

WILHELMINA (MINA) PÄCTHER, POET

 DO YOU EVER FEEL LIKE YOU NEED A LITTLE EXTRA encouragement with your eating struggles and dietary concerns? Ritual blessings can give you hope and something to hold onto, especially during the winter season when you may spend more time indoors.

It may help to remember that as difficult as your eating struggles may be, you are not alone. The above poem, for example, illustrates the determination of women who used poetry and recipes to help them survive confinement in a concentration camp. Know that you, too, can use ritual blessings to give you strength and courage at mealtime.

Feel free to recite your ritual mealtime blessing anytime you need it. Write it down and carry it with you so you can use it at any meal. Also, you may find that sharing it with another is also useful. You can share mealtime blessings just as easily as recipes.

♦

Use ritual blessing for extra encouragement
in your time of need.

Eating

When hungry I eat; when tired, I sleep. Fools
laugh at me. The wise understand.

ZEN MASTER RINZAI

MANY PEOPLE – BECAUSE OF SCHEDULES AND cultural norms – follow a three-meal-a-day routine. But what about those times your schedule frees you up, such as when you are on vacation or on weekends? And for those who have no enforced schedule, when should you eat?

Do not let enforced cultural habits hijack your body's natural rhythms. Eating only when you are hungry or to the level that satisfies your hunger is a more natural pattern. You may want to reexamine your three-meal-a-day routine and give yourself the space and permission to eat when you are really hungry.

If you work at home, for example, it does not make sense to force yourself to eat before your body signals you with appetite. Likewise, if you wait until you are famished and then overeat or eat unmindfully, then this strategy is not working! Always be mindful of your body's natural instincts.

◆

When your schedule is open, wait
for your body's appetite and subtle
signals before eating.

Community

To bring a person into your house
is to take charge of his happiness for as
long as he is under your roof.

ANTHELME BRILLAT-SAVARIN,
FRENCH GOURMET AND LAWYER

DO YOU EVER HAVE GUESTS OVER FOR DINNER or a cup of tea? This ancient ritual of hospitality and sharing of food and resources is thousands of years old. In some cultures, shared meals are a form of currency through which lifelong bonds and friendships are formed.

The next time you invite people to your dwelling to share food, think about how you can be mindful toward your guests. First, you can accomplish this by respecting and honoring guests with your full attention. Use kind speech that expresses what you genuinely feel – but only if it is beneficial and not self-serving. Lastly, listen to your guests by letting them share their unique stories – of their families, lives, or work.

In another sense, how you nurture others reflects how you nurture yourself. Naturally, remember to share your mutual love of food and drink.

✦

Invite guests over for a dish of
hospitality and mindfulness.

Departure

*I've been on a diet for two weeks
and all I've lost is two weeks.*

TOTIE FIELDS, PERFORMER AND COMEDIAN

DO YOU MONITOR YOUR WEIGHT FREQUENTLY?
Do you step on a scale at least once a day? If so, you might
consider doing the unthinkable – give that scale away or put it in
your closet.

By constantly checking your weight, you are focusing in on a
very limited aspect of your body and its relationship to food: You
are defining yourself by your weight. That may seem like the most
important thing at this moment, but the truth is that you cannot
measure who you are as a whole person by simple numbers. Your
waist size, your weight, your height, your shoe size, dress size, and
shirt size have no bearing on the story of who you are – unless you
let them.

Rather than focusing on the scale, observe your thoughts and
emotions around losing weight. Then, think how you can redefine
your relationship with weight loss.

◆

Make a choice to bring moderation and
compassion into your relationship with food
and weight loss.

Entry

*Approach a great painting as thou wouldst
approach a great prince.*

KOBORI-ENSHIU, TEA MASTER

DO YOU EVER APPROACH YOUR MEAL AS A WORK of art? Do you ever recognize the divine beauty, wonderment, and artistry that it represents? Or do you enter mealtime with apathy, indifference, fear, or another negative feeling?

Imagine how shifting your perception would change your mealtime experience. By preparing to approach your meal as you might "a great prince" you show that you understand the honor of your position and realize that you have been granted a sitting with the most divine nobility! (How cool is that?)

Naturally, you deeply respect the meal before you, share your secrets with it – by selecting that special diet of foods meant just for you. And in return, the "prince" – your meal – bestows upon you sublime gifts of life, energy, and well-being. It's a win-win. Enjoy it.

◆

Approach your meal with respect
due a divine prince.

Choices

So whenever your relationship is
not working, whenever it brings out the
"madness" in you . . . be glad.

ECKHART TOLLE, *The Power of Now*

DO YOU THINK ABOUT A FOOD AND IMMEDIATELY follow up by eating it? Does compulsive eating "madness" ever leave you wondering if your relationship with eating will ever have a positive outcome?

When thoughts about food are followed by what seems like an irresistible impulse, use what I call the "one-minute mindful time-out." As soon as you get a food impulse, breathe mindfully for one whole minute. Stay focused on your breath, even if you have intruding thoughts about that food. If possible, try to find a place to sit and take your one-minute mindful timeout. When you are done with your minute, you have built up strength-power and short-circuited the thought-eating impulses.

Stay with this practice and you can lengthen it over time from one minute to two minutes, and so on. Each time you do this, the impulse will weaken. The trick is to keep practicing!

◆

Use food madness to practice a one-minute
mindful timeout.

Preparations

One sits the whole day at the desk and appetite is standing next to me. "Away with you," I say. But Comrade Appetite does not budge from the spot.

LEONID BREZHNEV, FORMER SOVIET PREMIER

DOES YOUR APPETITE GROW STRONGER AS YOU prepare your meal? Does it affect how quickly you cook and what you decide to make for your meal? Do you hold your appetite at bay until you have finished preparing, or do you nibble as you cook?

As you undoubtedly know, Comrade Appetite does not easily budge, especially while you prepare your meal. What is important here is to be mindful of your appetite before you begin your preparations.

A strong appetite, for example, might prompt you to make a quick meal, a less than complete meal, or junk food so that you do not have to wait long before eating. But if you are mindful, then you can recognize the strength of your hunger while even making a meal that might take longer to cook.

✦

Be aware of Comrade Appetite before you
begin mealtime preparations.

Rituals

O Lord, as we now break the fast
We thank Thee for the night safe passed.
Now grant safekeeping on our way,
Good cheer and strength and health all day.

THOMAS ELWOOD, AUTHOR

DO YOU RUSH OFF IN THE MORNING WITHOUT A good meal? Is your need for food lost in your thoughts about the day ahead? If so, use a morning mealtime blessing to center you in relation to food for the remainder of the day.

Even if you eat a small breakfast, a blessing like the one above lets you acknowledge that you're breaking of the fast from the night before. (Few recognize that sleeping is also nature's way of fasting from food and drink to realign the body.) The blessing clues you and your body into the rhythm surrounding nourishment and eating. It makes you mindful that food is about your wellness and cannot be ignored – and that meals cannot be ignored.

This little morning blessing might trigger a thought later in the day that you need to take a break – that your body needs to take a break – for sustenance and recharging with a healthy meal.

◆

Use a morning blessing to bring
healthy eating into sharper focus for
the rest of your day.

Eating

*The food here is so tasteless you could
eat a meal of it and belch and it wouldn't
remind you of anything.*

REDD FOXX, COMEDIAN

DOES THE FOOD YOU EAT NEVER QUITE MEET your standards? Are you extremely picky and unhappy about the food you eat?

A friend of mine knows a woman who used to create a fuss every time she went to a restaurant. For example, she would send all her food back to be recooked and replaced – as well as the food of the people she was dining with! Not surprisingly, her dining partners dwindled in number until she got the message and began to deal with how she took out her general unhappiness on others, including the restaurants she frequented.

Are you mindful of how your reactions and emotions affect how food tastes as you eat it? Do you always find something lacking – not just in your food, but in your life and other relationships? If so, listen and observe more closely to your critical voice around food.

✦

Become more mindful of parallels between
how you eat and how you live.

Community

*A crust eaten in peace is better than
a banquet partaken in anxiety.*

AESOP

DO YOU EVER FEEL NERVOUS EATING WITH A GROUP OF people for the first time? Eating with a new family can leave you feeling uncertain about that group's style of relating to food. You may in fact be judged by how well you fit accepted eating standards.

I can remember, for example, eating dinner at the home of a family where no one took a second helping. I did not know this, of course, until I took my second helping – a normal occurrence in my own family. Of course, everyone looked at me as if to say, "Hey, you broke the rules!"

Many families have their own eating styles – such as eating fast or slow. If you are new to that group – or if you are already part of it and change the way you eat – then you may feel anxiety because you are breaking an ingrained custom. In addition, some groups may have dietary standards that do not meet your own requirements.

If this happens, you need to decide how to proceed – either to go along with group standards or to stick by your principles. Whatever you choose, you can be compassionate and accepting toward those who eat differently than you.

◆

Be accepting toward those with different
eating standards – even as you make your
own responsible choice.

Departure

Plenty sits still, hunger is a wanderer.

SOUTH AFRICAN PROVERB

HOW CALM DO YOU FEEL AFTER YOUR MEAL? Do you feel like the edge has been taken off your hunger? Or do you still feel unsatisfied and restless?

It is useful to be mindful of your appetite after eating. If you are still restless, for example, then this could be the result of drastically restricting your food intake to lose weight. I believe that losing weight does not mean forcing yourself to eat very little. Moderately eating healthy foods and being mindful of your eating habits still allows you to feel satisfied after mealtime.

Also, if you typically overeat, then even normal meal portions may leave you feeling dissatisfied and hungry. In this case you can (1) slow down your eating by breathing between bites, (2) chew more frequently, and (3) mindfully focus on the aroma, texture, and taste of food so that you are fulfilled by it, instead of just being filled up.

◆

Be mindful of whether you are restless
after mealtime, and take action to get
fulfilled rather than just filled up.

Entry

The two biggest sellers in any bookstore are the
cookbooks and the diet books. The cookbooks tell
you how to prepare the food and the diet books
tell you how not to eat any of it.

ANDY ROONEY, AUTHOR AND CORRESPONDENT

COOKBOOKS AND DIET BOOKS ARE OFTEN OPPO-
site one another in the same aisle of the bookstore. If you
struggle with emotions regarding your upcoming meal, then you
might find that this bookstore arrangement also perfectly reflects
your internal struggle over food.

Think about it. On the one hand you crave and desire food
badly; on the other hand you feel the need to control those urges
that threaten to take over your life and body. Is it possible for you
to let these apparently opposing desires coexist in peace?

By using mindfulness, you can be fully aware without being
pulled in both directions and beaten up by opposing thoughts.
Imagine yourself walking through the bookstore aisle with your
"cookbook thoughts" on one side and your "diet book thoughts" on
the other. Let yourself simply walk through the aisle without grab-
bing a "book thought" off the shelf.

◆

Enter your meal in peace by mindfully watching
your opposing thoughts and emotions.

Choices

One reason I don't drink is that I want
to know when I'm having a good time.

MAE WEST, FILM STAR

DO YOU EVER CHOOSE FOODS THAT LEAD TO mindless eating? Do you let your senses and emotions rule your dietary choices? Sometimes, mindless eating can be triggered by the foods you select.

Imagine that you are emotionally upset and about to choose food. Picture where you are: in the kitchen, car, or grocery store. In your upset state, what foods do you crave? What comfort food will temporarily improve your mood? From experience, reflect on whether this food choice leads to moderate or mindless eating.

You can mindfully intercept your food emotional choice. First, take a few relaxing breaths and feel your emotions. Name them by what they are: frustration, anger, disappointment, loneliness, etc. Next, visualize how you will feel after your mindless food choice, including how your stomach feels, as well as how you mentally and emotionally feel. Finally, give yourself permission to take care of yourself with a mindful, healthy choice.

◆

Intercept your mindless food choices by
becoming aware of your emotions.

Preparations

Simplicity is the mark of a master-hand.
Don't run away with the idea that it is easy to cook
simply. It requires a long apprenticeship.

ELSIE DE WOLFE, AUTHOR

DO YOU EVER WATCH COOKING PROGRAMS ON TV? Do you marvel at how easily the chef whips up almost any dish? But when you try to replicate the chef's actions at home, does the process feel awkward and complicated?

Most things that appear easy are the result of much practice and effort, and preparing food is no exception. It is not uncommon, for example, for professional chefs to begin their careers by chopping, dicing, and preparing foods for others who actually make the food. The chef who makes it look easy has probably done it hundreds of time – yet the excitement is still there.

The more you practice and find joy in cooking, the easier and simpler the preparation will be for you. If you only cook occasionally, be mindful of your skill level, and do not let frustration and expectation hamper your joy of cooking.

◆

Be mindful of your preparation skill
level and practice with joy.

Rituals

Hear me, four quarters of the world –
a relative I am! Give me the strength to walk the
soft earth, a relative to all that is!

BLACK ELK, HOLY MAN OF THE SIOUX

DO MEALS HELP YOU FEEL A SENSE OF KINSHIP with those around you? There are mealtime ritual blessings, like the one above, which can help you connect to all things – from the food on your plate to the people in your life.

If you feel alone in your eating struggles, a mealtime blessing that connects you with others can offer strength and encouragement. I remember, for example, when I took four Buddhist monks to lunch. After the meal, without warning, the monks chanted a short ritual blessing for all beings. The ripples of their chant spread positive energy throughout the restaurant. I think it might have made people feel more mindful and connected at that moment.

Whether it is before, during, or after your meal, the right ritual blessing can let others know you are a relative – through your words and actions.

◆

Use a mealtime ritual to awaken your kinship
with all others and offer you support.

Eating

Health food makes me sick.

CALVIN TRILLIN, JOURNALIST AND HUMORIST

DOES THE THOUGHT OF CERTAIN FOODS CAUSE you to react negatively? Do other foods make you feel joyful and excited? What you are experiencing is not really that unusual. That is because your emotional states can become linked to certain foods.

The next time you are in an emotional rut, become mindful of your impulse choices and what you avoid. Over time, certain foods can get associated with a mood or feeling. Suppose that when you feel down or physically ill you treat yourself to ice cream. Eventually, ice cream can elicit a positive mood. Conversely, food that may be healthy could have a negative association because of the situation in which you first encountered it.

As you taste food, mindfully observe your emotions – how they change. Then, consider varying your menu to force emotional issues that need dealing with to the surface.

◆

Be mindful of which foods and
moods go together.

Community

*A café is not a filling station for fueling the human
engine with a quick shot of caffeine; it is a way
station where travelers may dawdle for ten
minutes or three hours as their dispositions and
appointment calendars demand.*

JOSEPH MAZO, AUTHOR

 DO YOU EVER TAKE THE TIME FOR A LEISURELY meal with others? Or do you usually eat in front of the computer? Is your only purpose with eating to fuel your engine so you can get moving again? The emphasis on efficiency and multitasking in our culture has sapped mealtime's power to bring people into touch with others.

Drive-through espresso stands, fast-food restaurants, and convenience stores may feed you with a quick shot of energy, but they do little to fulfill you with human contact – which is another important purpose of food.

The point here is not to make every meal a social event. Rather, it is to acknowledge the need to slow down, digest the world around you, and find community through the most natural of means – food.

◆

Make the intention to meaningfully speak
with someone as you eat a meal.

Departure

*After a perfect meal we are more susceptible to the
ecstasy of love than at any other time.*

DR. HANS BAZLI

DO YOU FEEL MORE EMOTIONALLY AVAILABLE after a good meal? Do you find that you are more at ease, patient, and approachable? This may be especially true when you eat just the right amount – not too much or too little. No matter how perfect your meal, however, you cannot open to ecstasy if you do not take time to rest afterward.

State the intention to let yourself be emotionally at ease, content, and restful after your meal. When I visited Rome and Florence, for example, I was struck by how meals were never rushed – even in restaurants. Even after meals, people went outside and gathered near the beauty of timeless sculptures and fountains. They let their post-mealtime ecstasy open them to their surroundings.

You can do the same by walking outside. Find ecstasy in the walk, the company, and whatever else you may find.

◆

Experience ecstasy after your meal by taking
time to reflect and be open.

Entry

*The chief pleasure in eating does not consist in
costly seasoning or exquisite flavor, but in yourself.*

HORACE, *Satires*

WHAT IS YOUR ATTITUDE AS YOU PREPARE TO EAT today? Are you thinking about yesterday's eating fiasco? Are you fretting about your lack of control earlier in the day? Your thoughts and beliefs about food and eating have powerful consequences. The more you focus on your "mistakes," the more you may tend to repeat them.

The fact is that you can focus on the positive just as easily. I know a young lady, for example, who insisted that whenever she thought about peanut butter, she had to run out and get some. She did not realize that she had the control necessary to talk with me and not eat peanut butter until I pointed it out to her.

No matter how often you think you lack control, you do possess many good skills. You only need to become aware of them.

◆

Be mindful of the times throughout
the day when you are skillful in your food
actions and attitudes.

Choices

When you feel craving, you could be sitting on the edge of the Grand Canyon, but all you can see is this piece of chocolate cake that you're craving.

PEMA CHÖDRÖN, *Start Where You Are*

DO YOU EVER EXPERIENCE CRAVING SO STRONG that you lose sight of all other food choices? This narrowing of your choices is common when it comes to extreme cravings. I know someone who, when she has a food craving, needs to satisfy it within the next twenty-four hours. Is this also you?

Even when a craving becomes overwhelming, you can still be mindful of it. Let yourself feel the craving close up for as long as you can. One way to do this is to lie down and let it rest for a few minutes. Learn where you feel it in your body. Experience the images and thoughts it conjures from your past. See if you can determine under what circumstances it is most extreme.

The longer you can be mindful of your craving – by making it your friend – you will slowly begin to understand it. And, by not giving in immediately, you will be stronger the next time the craving appears.

◆

Experience your craving close up.

Preparations

On days when warmth is the most important
need of the human heart, the kitchen is the place
you can find it; it dries the wet sock, it cools
the hot little brain.

E. B. WHITE, AUTHOR AND HUMORIST

DO YOU NOTICE THAT PEOPLE OFTEN GATHER IN kitchens when there is a party? How comfortable are you in your own kitchen space? Does it feel familiar and warm? Or does is feel like someplace where a foreign language is spoken?

If you are not sure, take a walk through your kitchen. How relaxed and at home do you feel? Is the space open or cluttered? Is it clean and inviting? Are the walls and flooring bright or dark?

Now look in the cabinets and refrigerator. Are the food choices diverse, healthful, and fresh? Do the dishes and utensils express who you are as a cook? Are there any new cookbooks, as well as old and trusted ones?

Feel free to make changes to the décor, foods, and utensils. After all, this is your kitchen.

✦

Explore how you really feel about your
kitchen, then make changes.

Rituals

*Let's join hands in a circle, please. Now look
around the circle, recognizing and acknowledging
each of God's beautiful creations with us this day.*

REVEREND BOB BIDDICK

DO YOU EVER JOIN HANDS WITH OTHERS AROUND
your meal? Do you ever use a mealtime ritual to acknowledge the value of others? Ritual blessings such as the one above can
bring your family and others closer.

Yes, rituals often focus on your relationship to food and the
earth. But they can just as easily be used as an entrée to engender
closeness and to give everyone at your table a voice.

For example, the blessing by Reverend Bob Biddick could be
expanded in several ways. It could continue by having each person
express his or her personal blessing for the meal.

Or it could lead into the reading of a chosen scripture or poem.
Then, each present could reflect on the reading by expressing his/her
feelings about what it means for him/her as the others respectfully
listen, but do not judge or even discuss.

◆

Let ritual blessing unite your table with
respect and expression for all.

Eating

*If thou tastest a crust of bread, thou tastest
all the stars and all the heavens.*

ROBERT BROWNING

DO YOU TASTE YOUR FOOD, OR DO YOU GULP IT without really experiencing and savoring it deeply? If you taste your food without being afraid or anxious, then you will not gulp down your meal. This practice lets you mindfully experience those foods that you tend to overeat or restrict.

Set the intention: "May I experience my food with all my senses." Now, with your sight notice its color and texture. Let yourself sense its aroma. As you bite and chew, feel the hot or coldness of the food. Then, note to yourself if it tastes spicy, sweet, sour, salty, bitter, or pungent. Chew until the flavor disappears.

Before taking another bite, listen and observe your mind and thoughts. What are your feelings telling you about this food and your eating? Continue experiencing all sensations and emotions until you want to stop – not because of fear, but because you are no longer physically or emotionally hungry.

✦

Savor the flavor, sights, smells, and
sounds of today's meal.

Community

*Power is not manifested in the human being. True
power is in the Creator. . . . And we must continue
to understand where we are. And we stand
between the mountain and the ant.*

OREN LYONS, CHIEF OF THE ONONDAGA

DO YOU RELATE TO FOOD IN TERMS OF CONTROL
and power? Do you define your relationship with food as
something you either win or lose at? If so, then you are fighting a
battle with yourself. Food is not an enemy.

Let your community – your family, friends, and others – act as
a moderating force in your power struggle with food. Through
community, witness the bigger picture of how food nourishes and
brings people together. Let the community help you become less self-
involved with emotional food struggles and more other-involved.

One way to do this is to volunteer at community gatherings.
Recently, for example, I was invited to speak at a church service. I
arrived early and noticed that several members were working in
the kitchen. I didn't know why until afterward – when fresh squash
soup and bread were offered to all. It's not about power, but about
a healing relationship with yourself and others.

◆

Expand beyond control and power
and see the bigger picture.

Departure

*I am not necessarily wise and others are not
necessarily fools. We are all just ordinary men.*

Shotoku Taishi, prince of ancient Japan

WHEN YOU LEAVE YOUR MEAL, DO YOU EVER mentally defend your diet or approach to eating as being superior to what others eat? Attachment to your diet may limit your future choices and can be a contributing factor in keeping you from breaking addictive styles of eating.

Like clothing styles and fads, dietary fads also cycle in popularity. New diets bring the hope of changing your body shape, weight, waistline, and emotional outlook. However, many diets set unreasonable expectations that end up creating anxiety and doubt: "Is the diet working?" "Why am I not losing weight as quickly as the diet plan says?" "Why don't I look different yet?" Eventually, all your energy becomes caught in a web of exhausting emotional ups and downs.

Even if you stay on a diet, keep a balanced perspective. Most importantly, let go of your diet expectations.

◆

Do not become a slave to your diet. Do it for
good health and well-being – your body's
shape and weight will naturally follow course.

Entry

*Now as we become more conscious, we can see yet
more clearly the inevitable contradictions of
life . . . the ever changing play of joys and sorrows
that make up human experience.*

JACK KORNFIELD, *A Path with Heart*

THERE ARE MANY SITUATIONAL LIFE CHANGES that can bring joy or sorrow into your life. Do you find that joy or sorrow changes how you eat and feel about food?

The more you examine and become mindful of the root of your situational eating patterns, the more you will be able to avoid mindless eating. How does the joy of a positive relationship, a new place to live, or a personal victory affect your eating? Likewise, how does the loss of a significant relationship, loss of a job, or other personal loss alter your emotions, cravings, and appetite?

Look at the triggers in your life. Journal or make a mental note of your feeling and the situation surrounding compulsive eating. Be honest. You may not like to admit that your job, partner, or kids stress you out, but identifying your trigger may help keep you from reacting mindlessly.

✦

What triggers cause you to eat mindlessly
and compulsively?

Choices

*Strength is the capacity to break a chocolate bar
into four pieces with your bare hands – and then
eat just one of the pieces.*

JUDITH VIORST, POET

DO YOU HAVE THE STRENGTH TO EAT A LITTLE less (or more) for your overall health? Breaking a chocolate bar is easy. It's eating one piece that requires constant practice and effort.

Do you ever fool yourself into thinking that because you eat something good you can eat bad foods over which you have little willpower? The first way to build up strength over any food is to be honest.

If you cannot refrain from eating or buying your most tempting food, just accept that for the moment – without blame and shame. At least you have a starting point.

Now, you can work on refraining for five seconds or a minute longer than in the past. For example, take a breath before eating that food. Take two breaths, or three breaths. Eventually, the desire may pass while you are breathing. Eventually, you can choose freely to eat that food or not to eat it.

✦

Build strength by taking one
breath at a time.

Preparations

What, at this moment, is lacking?

ZEN MASTER RINZAI

Do you ever feel like you are missing something when you are preparing your meal? Maybe it is a missing ingredient, flavor, or nutritional balance? Maybe it is an emotional feeling that comes from missing someone who is not present with you during preparation?

As you prepare for today's meal, ask yourself: What is lacking? Make a mental note of what would make your process of preparation feel more whole and complete. This could, for example, even be the need for greater personal peace, quiet, and harmony that allows you to focus on cleaning the clutter and preparing a loving meal.

Once you identify what is missing, you can skillfully fill these gaps. Also, remind yourself that just because something is missing, this does not mean failure. Instead, accept your preparation with joy for what author Jack Kornfield calls your "ordinary perfection" that includes even the blemishes.

❖

Accept "what's lacking" with grace and as
part of your ordinary perfection.

Rituals

Why is this day different from all the rest?

JEWISH SEDER PRAYER BOOK

THE ABOVE PHRASE FROM THE SEDER, OR JEWISH Passover ritual meal, offers a potent reminder of how every day is precious. Do your ritual blessings help you cherish this day? Do they help you become more mindful of each day and its blessings?

It is easy to get caught up in the flow of days that become months, years, and a lifetime without savoring the God-given blessings in each of them. Why not use a ritual mealtime blessing to reveal the rich narrative story of your family or religious tradition? As is done in the Passover story, you may simply ask the question, "Why is this day different from all the rest?" to yourself or others at your dinner table.

You can also focus this question in a number of different areas. For example, you may ask, "How is my meal today different from all other days?" Or "How do I feel about the way my family – present and past – approaches food?"

◆

Ask yourself, "How is my relationship with food different today from all other days?"

Eating

At the end of every diet, the path curves
back toward the trough.

MASON COOLEY, APHORIST

DO DIETING RESTRICTIONS FRUSTRATE YOU? Do you find the food you eat on a diet to be incompatible with your lifestyle? Diets that restrict certain foods may not be a good lifestyle fit. A low carbohydrate diet, for example, might limit the amount of bread you can eat, when a sandwich is all that is available. When this happens, you may be frustrated eating what is not on your diet, and rightfully so.

If you feel guilt and blame yourself for losing control of your diet at today's meal, think again. It may be the diet – not you – that is to blame. Instead of having to cheat on your diet, realize that your diet may be cheating you. It may be cheating you out of balance in your food choices. It may be forcing you to stick to patterns of eating that are not practical given your routine, genetics, and nutritional needs.

◆

Be mindful of when a diet is not
practical or realistic for you.

Community

*In spite of everything, I still believe that
people are really good at heart.*

ANNE FRANK

ANNE FRANK WAS AN EXTRAORDINARY PERSON.
She held onto her ideals even when the situation looked bleak. Do you hold onto your positive feelings about yourself – even in the midst of your most discouraging food struggles?

During your life's food journey, you may have good reason to be disappointed in certain family and friends. Perhaps you have been judged, teased, blamed, or criticized in some way relating to food or body shape. At the same time, there are those who understand your journey and are there to support you and accept you as you are.

Now is a good time to shift your focus toward a community of people with whom you can share your food journey and find balance with eating. This can be a formalized group like Overeaters Anonymous or an informal group of friends who share concerns about food.

◆

Hold on to your positive feelings as you seek
out the company of compassionate others.

Departure

*As I relax my bladder, an image of rivers surfaces
in my mind. . . . I stand up and push the metal
lever down, hearing a rush of waters flush my
yellow offering into the bowels of the Earth.*

NINA WISE, PERFORMANCE ARTIST

DO YOU EVER FEEL SHAMED OR TURNED OFF BY your body's process of digestion and elimination? While at a meditation retreat, longtime meditator Nina Wise experienced shame regarding her body's process of elimination. This experience also had a positive benefit: It helped her explore her body's I-thou relationship with the earth. She realized that her digestive and waste process did not occur in a vacuum, but was part of a sacred cycle.

Reflect on Nina's words as you experience elimination. Your body cleanses and returns its by-products back to the earth. What is shameful about that? The process of elimination is part of being in balance and letting go. Think about how your intestines play a sacred role in your well-being. Be aware of how the foods you eat make it easier or harder for your intestines to digest and eliminate.

◆

Experience elimination, from your shame to
your sacred I-thou connection with the earth.

Entry

I was angry with my friend:
I told my wrath, my wrath did end.
I was angry with my foe:
I told it not, my wrath did grow.

WILLIAM BLAKE

DO YOU DENY YOUR EMOTIONS AROUND FOOD? Do you enter mealtime feeling withdrawn? Or do you enter mealtime filled with anger or anxiety? Any of these reactions can be a sign that unhealthy thoughts and emotions are blocking your food mindfulness. (Other obstacles to mindfulness are tiredness, restlessness, doubt, and sense craving.)

When this negativity occurs, you may feel unable to control your eating. The key at such times is to first take a breath, and then simply label what you are thinking and feeling as you approach your meal. If you are angry, for example, just mentally repeat the words "angry, angry, angry." If your inner thoughts say you are help-less, just label this process by repeating "thoughts of helplessness, thoughts of helplessness."

Labeling puts space between you and the feelings. It lets you observe them without judging yourself.

◆

Put space between you negative feelings
and thoughts by labeling them.

Choices

If you fail to plan, you plan to fail.

PROVERB

 HOW OFTEN DO YOU MISS A MEAL BECAUSE OF A situation at home or work? Skipped meals cause hunger, which in turn can cause mindless and hasty food selection.

My suggestion is to have a backup plan. This way, you can always eat food that energizes you. Sometimes, a backup plan means knowing your surroundings and what is available. For example, some fast-food restaurants feature salads.

Also, are you aware of the products being sold in nearby vending machines? I once took three-hour classes in a building with two vending machines. On the first day of class I learned that only one machine offered items such as cottage cheese and yogurt. I was aware my choices were limited and took that into account before going to class.

Lastly, you always have the opportunity to make (or buy) food and carry it with you.

◆

Plan ahead for skillful food choices.

Preparations

Do not make a stingy sandwich.

ALLAN SHERMAN, WRITER AND HUMORIST

 DO YOU PREPARE YOUR MEALS WITH AN OPEN heart? Do you buy enough food when you go to the store? Do you prepare your food so there will be enough on your plate – in both variety and quantity?

There are many ways to be generous in your preparation of food. First, you can be generous with your feelings and attitude toward cooking. You can experience cooking as an art and an expression of love – for yourself and others.

Next, you can be generous in your choice of ingredients and recipes. You can harmonize seasonal and local foods together. You can create a new recipe or experiment with a different combination of spices.

Finally, you can be generous in your quantity by making a little more than normal. Set the intention that you do not have to waste it or be compelled to eat it all. Instead, share it with others.

◆

Extend your generosity to preparation.

Rituals

I seek strength, not to be greater than my brother,
but to fight my greatest enemy – myself.

NATIVE AMERICAN PRAYER

DO YOU EVER FEEL STUCK IN REGARD TO YOUR food struggle? Do you feel like you are not gaining any new insights about why you eat the way you do? If so, then you may benefit from a ritual blessing that helps you gain strength, courage, and focus.

A ritual blessing like the one above puts any personal struggle in perspective. No one can be strong and in control all the time. It is natural that for every two steps forward you will take one step back. The journey of food is not a straight line. In your journey there will always be challenges and new things to learn.

Most importantly, be mindful of whether you are fighting others on this journey. Does fighting others get you closer to learning more about yourself – or does it just distract you? That is why a blessing for strength and self-knowledge is so important.

◆

Seek self-knowledge when you feel stuck.

Eating

What destroys craving?
Realization of one's true self.

SHANKARA, NINTH-CENTURY HINDU SAGE

DO YOU FEEL DRIVEN BY CRAVING WHEN YOU EAT? Do you eat ravenously? Are your cravings so strong that you feel helpless and unable to change them? The spiritual being within you transcends your cravings and desires, and you can use this knowing part of you to observe, accept, and heal them.

Food cravings and sense desires represent a powerful obstacle to maintaining mindfulness as you eat. (They are also an obstacle to spiritual growth, which is why observing them is important.) Food's flavor and taste can be so overwhelming that you may forget about everything else until you have overeaten and it is too late. Fortunately, you can break the hold of cravings by labeling them.

When you mentally label your sensations, you establish a momentary separation between yourself and the craving. While eating chocolate, for example, you might label your craving by mentally repeating, "desiring chocolate, feeling extreme hunger and craving, desiring more of the creamy texture and sweet flavor."

As you label your cravings, you can watch them rise and subside. And always, a mindful breath between bites helps.

◆

Label your cravings and
return to mindfulness.

Community

To the attentive, each moment of the year has its
own beauty, and in the same field it beholds, every
hour, a picture which was never seen before, and
which shall never be seen again.

RALPH WALDO EMERSON

DO YOU ACCEPT THE VARIOUS EATING FLAWS, frailties, and shortcomings that exist in your household, family, and community? Do you accept these or fight against them when they arise? Not only do disordered eating and emotions around food travel within you, they also travel across generations.

Have you noticed similar eating patterns, emotions, or issues around food that exist in the generations of your parents and grandparents? Sometimes these issues are not openly discussed. But you can look for clues. For example, is there a great emphasis on body weight and shape? Is there a history of obesity? Are you aware of unusual family stories around food or excessive exercise?

As you gain a broader picture of your family's eating style, do so with compassion and openness. Seek not to change them, but to behold the beauty and strength they possess – even in their struggle around food.

◆

Reflect on your family's journey around food.

Departure

A waist is a terrible thing to mind.

DAVE BARRY, SYNDICATED HUMORIST

DO YOU FREQUENTLY WORRY ABOUT YOUR WAIST-line? Do you compare your adult body shape to the body shape you had in your teens or twenties? I know of one middle-aged man, for example, who still makes comparisons with how much he weighed when he was in college. As you can imagine, he is never satisfied with his weight and body.

What weight and body standard do you hold yourself up to? Be mindful of the bodies that you watch on TV, magazines, and ads. Do they represent what is out there in the real world? I am not saying that you should not try to look and feel your best. But how realistic are your expectations? Do your expectations make you feel angry, disappointed, frustrated with yourself and your body?

The truth is this: Your body ages and changes. This is a natural process for all persons – and all living things.

◆

Be aware of your negative feelings
toward your body, then emotionally honor
your body by accepting and loving it.

Entry

Remember that happiness is a way of travel –
not a destination.

ROY M. GOODMAN, AUTHOR

HOW MUCH EMPHASIS DO YOU PLACE ON YOUR upcoming meal? Do you plan your day around it? Is eating your destination? Do not get me wrong – eating is important. After all, this book and many others are entirely devoted to it. Yet as vital and pleasurable as it can be, food's deeper purpose may be how it serves as a training ground for self-knowledge.

The mindfulness you apply as you approach a meal can be applied to other entry points in your life. As you explore your feelings around food, you can also investigate your feelings around any relationship. Being highly critical of how you eat and look, for example, could be one aspect of your inner critic. Does this inner critic, for example, also target boyfriends, girlfriends, and others who fail to meet "perfect" standards?

Do not take your food trip so seriously. Enjoy what you learn along the way.

◆

Let your next meal be an exploration of your
feelings, not a final destination.

Choices

*Almost every person has something secret
he likes to eat.*

M. F. K. FISHER, AUTHOR

DO YOU HAVE A SECRET FOOD OR SECRET EMO-
tional craving that drives your desire for food? Why is this
food/emotion a secret for you? Do you restrict a secret food choice
even though you like it intensely?

For example, my secret food is one that I rarely eat today, but
remember fondly from childhood – whipped cream. When our
parents were not around, my brother and I would shake the can
and spray the whipped cream right onto our hands. Sometimes we
would have a food fight with it. Today, however, it is not a food
choice for me. But should whipped cream adorn a dessert or hot
chocolate, I am never disappointed.

Sometimes, secret foods can be caused by secret emotional
cravings. It is okay to bring your secret foods and secret emotional
cravings into the light. When you do this, you remove any shame
or embarrassment surrounding them. Give yourself permission to
experience and enjoy your secret food in moderation.

◆

What is your secret food? Why do you feel
about it the way you do?

Preparations

The true cook is the perfect blend, the only perfect
blend, of artist and philosopher.
NORMAN DOUGLAS, *An Almanac*

DO YOU HAVE A CORE PHILOSOPHY ABOUT FOOD? Also, how does your food philosophy interact with your feelings about food and your food cravings? These questions can determine how you prepare your meals – or if you prepare your meals.

If you really think about it, your food philosophy may be central to your food struggles – including your feelings about preparation. There are many definitions of philosophy. My dictionary describes it from "love and pursuit of wisdom" to "the system of values by which one lives."

Do any of the following philosophies color your view of food preparation? Food is only necessary for survival. Food is the expression of love. The purpose of food is to bring people together. Food is medicine. Food is pleasure. Food is sin. Food is sacred.

Be honest in looking at your own food philosophy. Let yourself be flexible enough to choose more than one.

◆

Use your food philosophy to guide
today's meal preparation.

Rituals

And the drums will beat, and we will all dance.
Being a child is over – and I must start the dance
of womanhood – while the drums beat out my life.

ALICE PERRY JOHNSON, POET

DO YOU HOLD ON TO YOUR CHILDHOOD FEELINGS about food? Do you let past emotions around eating hurt you in the present moment? You can use a mealtime ritual blessing to invite a broader range of balanced thoughts and emotions into your life right now.

A ritual blessing like the one above acknowledges your intention to fully inhabit your present moment. Like a powerful rite of passage, it helps you to recognize old feelings as you take on new ones.

As you make this passage, you might want to ask, "What is my new dance around food?" Be mindful and aware of the new range of thoughts and emotions that you bring into your meals and life. At the same time, balancing out familiar emotions – even negative ones – can take time. So repeat this ritual blessing often as you heal and adjust to your new, healthy dance with food.

◆

What mature, healing emotions can you
invite to your rite of passage around food?

Eating

*He who distinguishes the true savor of his
food can never be a glutton; he who does not
cannot be otherwise.*

HENRY DAVID THOREAU

DO YOUR EMOTIONS EVER GET IN THE WAY OF tasting food? Do you get carried away by craving and lose your ability to discriminate between flavors? When you really savor food with mindfulness, one bite at a time, you are less likely to eat indiscriminately and to excess.

Hunger can hinder your ability to taste food, as well as cause you to eat quickly. First, rate your hunger on a scale of 1 to 10 (1 being no hunger and 10 being extreme hunger). Next, if your hunger is in the high range, take five mindful breaths to gain focus before you order or eat.

Then, recite a ritual blessing – even a short one – to give thanks for your meal and set your intention to eat mindfully.

Finally, taste one food on your plate at a time. Chew up to twenty-five times with each bite and observe how the flavor subtly changes.

◆

Be mindful of your hunger and take the effort
to savor each bite with mindfulness.

Community

Kindness is the key to men's work.

Confucius, *The Sayings of Confucius*

 Do you use food as a tool for expressing "living kindness"? Living kindness is the variety of ways by which you enthusiastically offer love, compassion, patience, generosity, wisdom, and truth to others. There is, perhaps, no better vehicle than that of food for providing opportunities for living kindness on a daily basis.

For example, here are some of the positive healing actions that you can take during your next family, household, or communal meal: Show generosity through food; enthusiastically support another's goals; be patient as you notice different eating styles; listen and speak gently; wisely eat a simple and wholesome diet; reveal your true authentic self; incorporate meaning with a ritual blessing; be resolute in your effort to eating mindfully; be even-tempered and nonjudgmental of those around you; and express loving kindness by being attentive and caring.

◆

See how many expressions of living kindness
you can bring to your communal meal.

Departure

*The Master gives himself up to whatever
the moment brings.*

LAO TZU

DO YOU EVER SURRENDER TO YOUR TIREDNESS after eating by taking a brief nap? Do you ever simply accept the emotions that follow a meal without trying to fight them? Sometimes, you gain greater control in your life by consciously being present in the moment – rather than fighting what is present and being focused only on the outcome.

Suppose, for example, that when you finish your dinner you feel upset that you ate two helpings of dessert. Usually, you spend the rest of the evening having an internal fight about those extra calories, your lack of control, etc. It only makes you more upset about your eating problem tomorrow.

Of course, you could just accept your thoughts and feelings in the moment – without judgment. Yes, you ate two helpings of dessert. You cannot change this, but you can surrender to your disappointment. You can find compassion and acceptance for yourself in the moment – this is your strength and the essence of mindfulness.

◆

Surrender to your after-meal physical
and emotional feelings. Find your strength
in your compassion.

Entry

My stomach serves me instead of a clock.

JOHNATHAN SWIFT, EIGHTEENTH-CENTURY
ENGLISH NOVELIST AND POET

BEGINNING WITH THANKSGIVING DAY AND continuing through Christmas and New Year's Day, food seems to be everywhere. How do you navigate the deep-dish pumpkin pie, homemade cookies, chocolate kisses, fresh muffins, and free food tasting at the store? If you do not have a plan, you can be pretty stressed out and miserable by the end of the holiday season.

Fortunately, by being mindful of your real hunger, you will not have to follow an extreme diet plan come January 1. A good place to start is to be mindful of your past holiday eating patterns and frustrations.

For example, do you maintain control until Aunt Annie hands you her home-baked cookies – even though she knows you are trying to avoid them? You cannot change the Aunt Annies in your life. You can, however, bring the power of mindfulness to the situations you have faced many times before.

✦

Reflect on how you will use mindful eating
throughout the holidays.

Choices

*A piece of rope remains a rope, whether or not
we mistake it for a snake.*

SHANKARA, CREST-JEWEL OF DISCRIMINATION

 DO YOU HAVE STRONGLY HELD IDEAS ABOUT your food choices? Are some foods always good and others always bad? Do you, for example, turn that piece of cake into a snake? When a food becomes bad, then whoever eats that food, including you, also becomes bad. This kind of righteousness leads to blame and shame.

There are more balanced ways to view food choices. You can explore them by how they contribute to the harmony of your mind-body-spirit. Do you feel lighter or heavier? Do you feel more peaceful and calmer or anxious and agitated? Do you feel focused or distracted? This way you label food by its effect, and not by making it bad in itself.

Balance also means not having to deny and reject a food outright. There may be a time or place for a food in your life, without blame or shame. This Thanksgiving season, you can be less judgmental about food as you seek more balance and peace with food.

♦

Don't judge food or yourself harshly.

Preparations

This morning I ask only
The blessing of the crayfish,
The beatitude of the birds;
To wear the skin of the bear
In my songs;
To work like a man with my hands.

JOSEPH BRUCHAC, NATIVE AMERICAN
STORYTELLER AND AUTHOR

DO YOU LIKE THE FEEL OF WORKING WITH FOOD? Do you get a sense of satisfaction as you clean food and get your hands wet in the sink? Do you enjoy rubbing seasoning onto your food? That is no surprise, since food preparation is a powerful means of becoming grounded and centered with life. Like any work you do with your hands, food preparation is creative and practical.

Do not pretend that food preparation is at the fringe of eating a meal – a necessary chore to get out of the way as quick as possible.

On the contrary, it is your first taste and inner knowing of the sacredness of food. Let yourself become one with the work of preparation. Immerse yourself. Mindfully observe the transformation of food and you may observe your own transformation!

✦

Experience the power of being
grounded and centered through preparing
food with your hands.

Rituals

The deeper that sorrow carves into your being, the
more joy you can contain....
Some of you say "Joy is greater than sorrow," and
others say, "Nay, sorrow is the greater."
But I say unto you, They are inseparable.

KAHLIL GIBRAN, *The Prophet*

 DO YOU EVER GROW WEARY OF YOUR FEELINGS of sadness and anger around food? Do you ever wish you could forget them and have only happy thoughts and feelings? Words like those of Kahlil Gibran can be used as part of a ritual blessing to give you hope that while sadness exists, it is inseparable from joy.

As holidays like Thanksgiving come along, traditional blessings focus only on what you can be thankful for. Why not also be thankful for the emotions and the struggle that each meal brings? If this seems odd, consider that your struggle with food is helping you understand yourself more than the average person without a food issue.

Your food struggle gives you the blessing of mindfulness and savoring each bite. It helps you slow down, make more skillful choices, and reach out to others. These joys are no small accomplishments!

✦

Give thanks even for your sorrows and the
joy that springs from them.

Eating

Enough is as good as a feast.

JOHN HEYWOOD, SIXTEENTH-CENTURY WRITER

WHEN THE FOOD YOU ARE EATING IS GOOD, MORE food seems like a good idea. But when is enough food really enough? How do you know when you are about to go over the line?

At some point while you are eating, you may feel the impulse or desire to eat more. (This impulse can occur at any time, even when you are not eating.) When this happens, you can accept your impulse and thought in the moment without immediately acting on it. Just experience how it makes you feel – frustrated, upset, etc.

Second, be mindful of the actions you can take. Mentally state (or write down) the possibilities, such as: "I can leave and not take another bite. Or I could take one more bite, eat until I am full, or binge on food/candy bars/cookies, etc."

Lastly, take a mindful breath as you state your intention. At the same time, visualize the action you decide upon, and then follow through. Observe your feelings as you take action. You can also breathe mindfully for one minute, during which the impulse often lessens or fades away completely.

◆

Put the brakes on your impulse by
taking mindful action.

Community

Where the guests at a gathering are well-acquainted,
they eat 20 percent more than they otherwise would.

EDGAR WATSON HOWE, AUTHOR

DO YOU FEEL OBLIGED TO EAT MORE WHEN YOU are part of a festive gathering? Holidays are a difficult time to moderate food intake because so many festivals are celebrated and expressed with food. To deny food is to deny you are joining in. Fortunately, there are several good strategies for moderate holiday eating.

First, make it a practice to leave some food on your plate and eat slowly. Second, practice *statio*, a momentary pause prior to the main meal. In this way you do not deny yourself appetizers, but wait until the entrée is served before you eat any food. Third, be mindful of your liquor consumption, because too much alcohol may reduce your overall mindfulness about food. Finally, set the intention of how much you want to eat and drink before you go – so you will be mindful from the start of the festivities.

Also, take stock of those emotions that you tend to feel around the holidays. Be mindful of when they appear so you can keep emotional eating in check.

◆

Be aware of your party eating habits.
Set an intention before you go and then
enjoy yourself in moderation.

Departure

Garbage becomes rose.
Rose becomes compost –
Everything is in transformation.
Even permanence is impermanent.

THICH NHAT HANH

Do you ever marvel at how food transforms? It goes from being something that is separate from you before the meal into something that is part of you after the meal. This miracle is part of the continuing lesson on transformation that you – and all persons – receive through food and eating.

Since food becomes part of you, does it not also follow that you become part of it? It is critical that you understand this, because it helps you know how food can directly affect the way you feel. If you have a history of depression or hyperactivity, for example, there may be a connection to your diet – in particular, excess sugar.

Finding balance and harmony in life requires finding that same balance in your dietary choices. Eating sugar, carbohydrates, or any food to excess could affect you adversely. Change your diet (with medical supervision) and see if your moods improve and your cravings diminish.

◆

Change your diet to change your mood.

Entry

Least effort is expended when your actions are
motivated by love, because nature is held together
by the energy of love. When you seek power and
control over other people, you waste energy.

DEEPAK CHOPRA, *The Seven Spiritual Laws of Success*

HOW DO YOU FEEL WHEN YOU TRY TO CONTROL
your eating? Do you ever get tired of forcing yourself to
stick with a diet? Do you sometimes grow weary of counting calories? The truth is, it takes a tremendous amount of mental energy
to control eating. No wonder so many dieters feel fatigued and
exhausted.

On the other hand, you can let go of your power trip over your
own mind-body and let your actions be "motivated by love," as
Deepak Chopra wisely advises. For example, what if you relinquished the chains of control and instead channeled your energy into
being mindful of the love that exists in your life around food.

Be mindful of how food expresses love for your health and consciousness. You can also change your attitude toward the foods you
struggle with, such as moving from hatred and disgust toward an
attitude of love and acceptance. Motivated by love, you can choose
to stop fighting food at this moment and this meal.

◆

Shift your energy from controlling your diet
to love for yourself and others at mealtime.

Choices

Never buy sushi from a vending machine.

ANONYMOUS

DO YOU EVER GET FRUSTRATED HAVING TO EAT food that you do not really want? Do you ever end up with vending machine food because other choices simply are not available? These situations may force you to eat other foods – and perhaps less desirable foods. When this happens, it is important to be mindful of your feelings.

When you do not get your first choice, do you become angry, frustrated, or even depressed? How do these feelings trigger your next food selection? Be aware, for example, if you decide to numb your frustration by impulsively choosing a comfort food. Or you may use this situation as an excuse to eat something "bad" because you have no other options.

Remember that your karma is in your refrigerator, the vending machine, and your next food choice. Do your best to create a backup plan for those times that you cannot eat what you want. If you are not satisfied with what is available, you can always fast until a nourishing meal is available. Always be mindful of your emotions and make your choice a wise and patient one.

✦

Be mindful of how you feel when the food
you want to eat is not available.

Preparations

Some people's food always tastes better than others,
even if they are cooking the same dish at the same
dinner. Now I will tell you why – because one
person has more life in them – more fire, more
vitality, more guts – than others.

Rosa Lewis, English society caterer

Can you tell when a particular person cooks a meal just by tasting it? Is there someone in your life whose food transcends the ordinary? Extraordinary meals begin with their preparation.

Chefs who prepare exceptional food first season their preparation with love – the love of cooking, the love of food's flavors and aromas, the love of presentation, the love and thrill of creating something artistic, and the love of giving joy to others.

Negative emotions during preparation put bitter seasoning into the sauce. When you carry unhealthy emotions with you into the kitchen – jealousy, envy, hate, anger, boredom, etc. – they inevitably show up in the final product. How can you pay attention to the details of a meal when your thoughts and emotions are clouded and preoccupied?

If you feel negative emotions, pause, take a short walk, and come back to the kitchen when you can center yourself in loving thoughts.

◆

Be mindful of your negative emotions,
and season all your meals with love.

Rituals

God help us to live slowly:
To move simply:
To look softly:
To allow emptiness:
To let the heart create for us.
Amen.

MICHAEL LEUNIG, WRITER

DO YOU FIND THAT YOU GET MORE STRESSED out about food around the holiday season? Do you ever feel like you do not have time to slow down, let alone enjoy a meal? If so, you may want to incorporate a blessing like the one above into your mealtime.

When you "live slowly," you slow down and savor each bite of your meal, instead of worrying about future plans.

When you "move simply," you set a mindful intention to move with full presence and purpose amid the whir and bustle of others.

When you "look softly," you gaze without judgment and with compassion at those who feed themselves however they can.

When you "allow emptiness," you find space to be at peace with your own hunger even when confronted by temptation.

◆

Let your heart create a new season for all.

Eating

Life would be an easy matter
If we didn't have to eat.
If we never had to utter,
"Won't you pass the bread and butter."

NIXON WATERMAN, *If We Didn't Have to Eat*

DO YOU EVER WISH THE HOLIDAY SEASON HAD a little less emphasis on food and eating? Do you think your life would be easier without that "appetite" and "food issue" being tempted more than usual?

It helps if you appreciate and accept that holidays are for sharing and giving and receiving love and good cheer. Holiday food – with its special preparation and presentation – is an important material expression of that spirit. At this level, you can mindfully fill up on the caring intention of food and not the material expression of it.

Before eating, consciously state, "I can fill myself up on the intention of spirit and love that resides in this food." Next, recall a time when you skillfully tasted just enough of something and were satisfied by it. Then use the three mindfulness tools – your sensations, your mind/perceptions, and your body – to eat moderately. As you eat food, remember to breathe between bites and use that time to reflect on the spirit and love in the food you eat.

◆

Bring mindfulness tools and realistic
expectations to the holidays.

Community

*A host is like a general: it takes a mishap
to reveal his genius.*

HORACE, PHILOSOPHER

IMAGINE THAT YOU ARE ABOUT TO HOST A VERY special party. What feelings and expectations arise? Do you worry about the menu and the food being perfect? Do you feel your gathering must be more extravagant than someone else's party? No matter how much you plan, do you still worry even as the party is in progress?

One way to relax and enjoy your meal and guests is this: Surrender to the uncertainty of the moment. When you mindfully give in to the moment you release your expectations, fears, and hopes about the way things ought to be. Instead, you live with the way things are right now.

With mindfulness, your purpose is simply to share this moment and be attentive to those you care about. When you welcome uncertainty you also welcome spontaneous joy and laughter. You welcome the unique, unusual, and memorable into your life.

◆

Let go of expectations and invite others to
surrender with you to joyful uncertainty.

Departure

Hearty laughter is a good way to jog internally
without having to go outdoors.

NORMAN COUSINS, AUTHOR

WHAT IS YOUR MOOD AFTER EATING? DO YOU get anxious that you ate too much (or too little)? Do you feel heavy and weighted down because of what you ate? Do you go right from eating to intense physical or mental activity? If you experience pronounced moods or feelings such as these, then you could benefit from a gentler mealtime transition.

A skillful departure is essential to experiencing emotional joy and balance with eating. Eating is a time of enjoyment, so why not (en)lighten your departure with a transition of laughter and bliss?

For example, take a short walk and note all the pleasant things around you – clouds in the sky, children playing, a rose bush, fresh air, your own sense of wellness. Also, make pleasant conversation with another, read a few engaging pages in a favorite book, enjoy a cup of tea. By focusing on the positive, you block out negative feelings and create a healthier thought pattern.

◆

Lighten your mealtime departure with a few
moments of joy and laughter.

Entry

The greatest success is successful self-acceptance.
BEN SWEET, AUTHOR

DO YOU SOMETIMES HEAR A CRITICAL VOICE when you think about your next meal? Specifically, what does your inner critic say? Is it loudest before, during, or after your meal? When does it become quieter?

With self-acceptance you can witness yourself as not being defective, but as the whole being you are – and that includes both your skillful and unskillful thoughts and behaviors around food.

Unskillful and limiting thoughts fit some common categories. For example, all-or-none thinking might sound like this: "I'll never control my eating." There is self-blaming thinking: "It's my fault that I didn't eat a balanced meal." Another thinking category is misery-making: "Going to that dinner party is going to be a big mistake." There is guilty thinking: "I knew I shouldn't have had that second helping."

Since there are two sides to every thought, see if you can broaden your limiting thoughts. Over time, have faith that you can cultivate a more balanced voice that leads to self-acceptance.

◆

Hear and accept unskillful thinking patterns
as the first step of self-acceptance.

Choices

*The longer I work in nutrition, the more
convinced I become that for the healthy person all
foods should be delicious.*

ADELLE DAVIS, AUTHOR AND HEALTH AUTHORITY

HOW DO YOU DEFINE HEALTHY FOOD? DO YOU think healthy food tastes better (worse) than most other food? When you think about choosing a healthy meal, what is the first idea that pops into your head? As Adelle Davis suggests, there is no reason for healthy meals not to taste good.

Actually, you may be surprised to learn that many so-called ordinary good-tasting foods offer extraordinary health benefits. Peanuts, almonds, and other nuts are excellent sources of fiber that help food move through your digestive system. Whole-grain cereal is another ordinary food that contains a lot of fiber (although watch the sugar). The average tomato and watermelon contain a compound that combats prostate cancer. The common apple has been shown in studies to be good for the lungs. It also contains pectin, which helps to reduce cholesterol.

Make an effort to taste healthy food and learn more about what foods and substances support your health and which ones stress it.

◆

Balance your diet with healthy foods by
making an effort to learn more about them.

Preparations

*Every morning must start from scratch, with
nothing on the stoves — that is cuisine.*

FERNAND POINT, CHEF

WHEN YOU PREPARE YOUR MEAL, DO YOU START from scratch? By that, I mean, do you start with a clean slate? This suggests not just fresh foods, but a fresh and uncluttered mind, as well as a clean workspace.

To start with "nothing on the stoves" not only means cooking from scratch, but leaving past cooking mishaps behind. The beauty of mindful preparation is that you can enter the present whether you clean a countertop, scrub a potato skin, dice an onion, or rinse out a pot. Now is your chance to try a new recipe or become more skillful with an old one.

Use the mindfulness of body to pay attention to how you stand at the cutting board, how your fingers hold the knife, and how you stand and move about the kitchen.

As you work with food, use mindfulness of sensations to guide you as you taste, touch, and smell your creation.

Use mindfulness of awareness and perception to listen to your mind and perceptions and judgments as you cook.

Finally, open the space for silence, just to be aware of the wonder of it all.

◆

Start preparing from scratch,
uncluttered and mindful.

Rituals

*Let no one deceive another. Let no one despise
another in any situation. Let no one, from
antipathy or hatred, wish evil to anyone at all.*

THE BUDDHA

EATING IS A VERY HONEST ACT. FUNDAMENTALLY,
eating is about your body needing nourishment for which
food provides energy and well-being. There is no deception. When
you eat something, your body knows when that food is healthy
and beneficial, and it knows when you are trying to fool it!

Do you ever try to deceive your body (with your mind) by telling
yourself that an eating habit or food is really okay? I know a man,
for example, who once ate almost an entire carrot cake instead of his
regular dinner. The next day he was still feeling ill from the effect
of ingesting so much sugar and butter.

Just as a mother naturally loves her children, you need to love and
protect your own well-being. If you need help, recite the ritual blessing above by adapting it as "Let me not deceive my body."

◆

Be honest about eating at today's meal.

Eating

Some will receive their meal early in the morning,
others at noon, still others not until evening. But
none will go hungry. Without any exception, all
living beings will eventually know their own true
nature to be timeless awareness.

RAMAKRISHNA, HINDU SAGE

 WHAT DO YOU RECEIVE FROM YOUR MEAL AS YOU eat? There are many different layers of meaning for how you can taste today's meal.

As you sit down to eat today make a note of how your meal feeds you. For example, you can: Eat for your taste buds; eat for your self-image; eat to please others; eat for your emotions; eat for distraction; eat for self-control; eat for loss of control; eat for love; eat for attention; eat for pity; eat for self-blame; eat for your body's hunger; eat for security; eat for survival; eat for your mind's craving and sense desire; eat for energy and long life; eat so you have the energy to go and reduce the suffering of others; eat to gain self-knowledge of your own true nature and to be timeless awareness.

There is no right or wrong receiving. However you receive food today will lead to greater self-knowledge and peace.

◆

Discover the ways you receive your meal.

Community

*We have only begun to know the power that
is in us if we would join our solitudes in the
communion of struggle.*

DENISE LEVERTOV, POET

Do you ever feel alone in your struggle
with food? Do you find it difficult to share your food issues? Do you keep your struggle a secret?

In truth, the struggle with food is a universal one shared by communities across lines of gender and culture. The Bible's story of the
forbidden apple is echoed, for example, in the Buddhist creation
story – where angels taste a food so tempting that they end up
hoarding and fighting over it. Eventually, the unhealthy emotions
of greed, envy, jealousy, and lust destroy their angelic powers and they
fall to Earth and become human.

Your food issues only mean that you are experiencing the core
condition of all humans: how to bring the spiritual and physical
sides of your being into peaceful coexistence. The next time you
eat with others, let this perspective give you compassion for how
all people confront this in different ways – either through food,
work, sex, drugs, or other struggles.

◆

Know that your food struggles are universal
and very human.

Departure

Pause, reflect, choose, be aware, and be free.

DONALD ALTMAN

 DO YOU FOLLOW THE SAME ROUTINE AFTER MEALS? Do you leave dinner and immediately turn on the TV? It is easy to follow a routine because it is safe, secure, and predictable. On the other hand, it can keep you from engaging in other exciting options. How do you use the energy you take from eating?

Food can fill space and time, but you can do that by engaging in life (also a good antidote for evening snacking).

Begin with a pause after your meal. A pause is a moment filled with unlimited potential! No decision has been made. As you take a pause, take a long calming breath.

Next, reflect on what you could do at this moment. Is there a book to read? A friend to visit? A movie to see?

Now, choose the activity that you are prepared to undertake at this moment and how your energy lets you feel about yourself. Be aware of the thoughts, expectations, judgments, and obstacles that come into your mind. Then, do it anyway and be free!

◆

Break free of routine and engage in
something new after your meal.

Entry

Gave up spinach for Lent.

F. SCOTT FITZGERALD

Do you ever negotiate when it comes to eating more (or less)? For example, when you enter a restaurant and see a thick slice of pie (your favorite flavor), do you make a deal with yourself to eat a smaller lunch so you can have your dessert?

When you negotiate with your eating, are you really just giving up spinach for Lent? Fortunately, you have mindfulness of your mind and perceptions to clarify this.

Be mindful of your thoughts beginning with the moment you see the cheesecake. What is your inner dialogue? Often you may hear competing thoughts, such as, "I want that cheesecake, it looks fantastic!" and "I can't eat that, I've been trying to cut down on sugar."

Listen carefully to learn the truth if you are negotiating a deal because the craving is too strong. Even if you still choose to eat the cheesecake, at least you can be fully aware of your choice.

◆

Use mindfulness to shed light on how you
negotiate your eating.

Choices

Yesterday's kitchen is today's medicine.

MONIKA WOOLSEY, DIETITIAN

 HOW DO YOU DESCRIBE YOUR FOOD CHOICES? Do simple, basic foods appeal to you? Do you prefer foods that have been fried, processed, and smothered in sauce? Or do you like a combination of basic and complex foods depending on the situation?

There is no right or wrong answer to these questions. But know that a more simple diet probably fed most of your ancestors. A century ago, for instance, Americans ate very little sugar in their foods.

One example of a salad I enjoy from time to time consists of tomatoes, red bell pepper, onions, avocado, cucumber, garbanzo beans, a hard-boiled egg, feta cheese, and oil and vinegar dressing. It is an entire meal – one that contains basic, unprocessed ingredients and is easy to prepare. It is also filling and leaves me feeling light and energetic.

The point here is to find balance between complex and simple foods. Be open to the joy of a fresh apple off the tree. Be moderate with the gravy and sauces.

◆

Bring a balance and harmony of simplicity
into your food choices.

Preparations

If you want to make an apple pie from scratch,
you must first create the universe.

CARL SAGAN, AUTHOR

DO YOU EVER FEEL STRESSED AND OVERWHELMED in the kitchen around the holidays? Do you feel that baking an apple pie or cooking a whole turkey requires some special talent or apprenticeship? I must admit that while growing up there was a mystique around that holiday turkey that got carved up at family dinners.

Fortunately, as Carl Sagan writes, you are not really making an apple pie, or anything else, from scratch. This extends to family and friends whose love and good cheer are the expression of long-time caring relationships. You just have to set the stage and allow its natural expression to arise.

In other words, you don't have to orchestrate everything and everybody. Relax, the cakes will rise, the turkeys will cook, and good cheer will abound. If you find yourself starting to feel overwhelmed, slow down and take a mindful breath. Remember that you've been preparing for this holiday celebration all your life.

So smile. (En)lighten up. Cook the meal, not yourself.

◆

Bring joy and laughter into your holiday
kitchen and preparation.

Rituals

Forgive us our sins against Earth,
As we are learning to forgive one another.
And surrender us not unto extinction,
But deliver us from our folly.

HENRY HORTON

DO YOU HAVE A HOLIDAY FOOD FOLLY? WHERE does your folly lead you on the scale of blame and acceptance? A ritual blessing like the one above is one way to bring a broader perspective and forgiveness into your life, as well as your food folly.

Forgiveness is an important holiday theme, and it is one that you can explore during this month. Consider this: The winter season brings the end of a long cycle of planting, growing, and enjoying the fruits of your harvest. As the ground grows cold (or less warm, depending on where you live), your heart does not have to grow bitter or weary for the food follies you may have endured.

Have faith, for there is another season/day/meal just around the corner. Each new moment is the perfect place to be mindful. To plant the seed of awareness just by observing – without judgment – is a form of forgiveness in itself!

✦

Plant new seeds of forgiving at mealtime –
and anytime.

Eating

*Great food is like great sex – the more you have
the more you want.*

GAEL GREENE, FOOD CRITIC

DO YOU EVER LOOK AT A BANQUET TABLE FILLED with food and want to gobble it all up? Welcome the club of those whose eyes are bigger than their stomachs. Managing your food portions can be challenging – especially at an event where the food is plentiful and delectable.

It is easy to slip into mindless eating. First, you can lose your mindfulness when your craving or hunger is so strong that you start eating and cannot stop. A snack between meals might help you from being mugged by your appetite.

Emotional overload is another cause of mindless eating. If you feel emotionally overwrought, unhappy, or stressed, then you can use food to medicate yourself. Being mindful of your emotional state, such as noting, "I am stressed and sad and eating will make me feel better," can put the brakes on. Then, you consciously eat well, knowing that in the long run you will feel better with this decision.

◆

Be mindful of what can derail your eating.

Community

*Let thoughts of boundless love pervade the whole
world . . . without any hatred, without any enmity.*

THE BUDDHA

LOVE IS EASY TO TALK ABOUT, HARDER TO PUT into action. For example, do you ever wonder how you can express love at holiday mealtime gatherings? Generosity is a wonderful way to put love into action, and there are many flavors of mealtime generosity that you can be mindful of applying.

You can be mindful of giving others a voice at the table. Let them talk, share, and express what is in their hearts and minds without being judgmental.

You can be mindful of giving your time and effort by helping prepare the food, set the table, and clean up afterward.

You can be mindful of sharing by bringing food, drink, or dessert to accompany the meal.

You can be mindful of your patience by being attentive, serving others at the table, and waiting your turn to eat.

You can be mindful of loving kindness by showing your gratitude.

◆

Be mindful of how generous
you are at mealtime.

Departure

It often happens that I awake at night and begin to
think about a serious problem and decide I must
tell the pope about it. Then I wake up completely
and remember that I am the pope.

POPE JOHN XXIII

DO YOU EVER FEEL YOU HAVE TO SHARE YOUR serious problem around food with someone important? Do you ever stop to think that maybe you are that most important person, the one in charge and with all the answers?

True, there is a lot of food wisdom and guidance to be gained from others. There are wise sages, nutritionists, friends, therapists, family members, doctors, and so on. But there is only one expert who has been with you from day one and who knows you more intimately than anyone: you.

You are the master of your life and you determine – through your effort and skill and commitment – how you will use food. Ultimately, whether you use food for health, pleasure, medication, control, or love is your decision. Just watch. Be mindful of your emotions. Like the pope, you can wake up and start right now.

◆

Wake up and know that you are the
expert in your life.

Entry

The mystery is what's important.

JOSEPH CAMPBELL, MYTHOLOGIST AND AUTHOR

DO YOU EVER FEEL A SENSE OF MYSTERY AND wonderment about your next meal? Do you greet your upcoming meal with anticipation and excitement – just as you might when meeting your very best friend? What is your relationship with food right now, today?

Joseph Campbell, for example, believed that simple definitions of the divine could not really touch the mystery of God and transcendence that people really experience. Likewise, it is easy to get caught up in defining yourself by the diet you follow rather than the infinite mystery of your relationship with food.

The diet you follow is like a two-dimensional line drawing. How food enriches your life, how it shapes your interactions with others, how you use it to nourish mind-body-spirit, and how it connects you with the sacredness of life and emotions is a multidimensional, moving picture.

Just take it all in without trying to change it. Do not try to explain it. Just be with it and let it be.

◆

Rest in the mystery of your
relationship with food.

Choices

Parsley
Is gharshley.

OGDEN NASH, ENGLISH POET AND HUMORIST

EMOTIONS CAN RUN HIGH DURING THE HOLIDAYS. Do your feelings during family or other meals prejudice you to favor some foods and avoid others? Surely, there are traditional holiday foods you adore and others you abhor. Because family gatherings can sometimes be emotionally charged events, food can be the lightening rod that draws your emotions.

When your emotions become strained, do you fall back on prior eating patterns? If your family eats fast and you have learned to slow down, for example, how do you keep your own pace? At such times you need to be especially aware and mindful of your breathing, sensations, and emotions.

Most importantly, let yourself be the person you are now at your family holiday meal. You do not need to reassume the role of a child, teenager, or any other position you once filled. Eat what pleases you at holiday meals, but watch out for unreasonable expectations.

◆

Do not let food be the lightening rod
for your emotions.

Preparations

A lovely thing about Christmas is that it's
compulsory, like a thunderstorm, and we all
go through it together.

GARRISON KEILLOR, AUTHOR AND HUMORIST

DO YOU FIND THAT PREPARING A MEAL AT CHRIST-
mastime is like being in a thunderstorm? Or maybe it is
more like a hurricane. Naturally, there may be more than the usual
number of interruptions while preparing a meal that often has
many courses and more than one cook.

You may find it necessary to shift your focus while preparing a
large meal. In order to stay mindful, you can mentally state a new
intention each time you are called away to tend something else.
When you return to the previous task, again state your intention
to peel the potatoes, set the table, or whatever you were doing.

By restating your intention, you bring full attention back to your
work and can follow through instead of having your mind skip
from task to task and leading you around without getting a lot
done.

✦

State and restate your intentions to stay
on track as you prepare.

Rituals

Men go abroad to wonder at the heights of
mountains, at the huge waves of the sea, at the long
courses of the rivers, at the vast compass of the
ocean, at the circular motion of the stars, and they
pass themselves by without wonder.

St. Augustine, fourth-century saint

 Do you have a personalized mealtime ritual blessing? If not, what unique aspect of your personal life story could one contain? What strengths could it help you to tap into?

I have facilitated others creating their mealtime blessings, and I am always awed at the results. Create a ritual blessing alone or with others. It is sometimes helpful to divide into two person teams to brainstorm.

For the blessing portion of your ritual blessing, use your own words, as well as other wise sources like scripture, poetry, people, and books of prayers. As themes, consider balance, the hero's journey, initiation, justice, love, peace, strength, empowerment, healing, growing old, sharing, mindfulness, and praise for the earth.

The ritual portion could be any action from holding hands and lighting a candle to singing and creating a sacred space around which to say your blessing.

◆

Create a meaningful blessing and ritual
to share with others.

Eating

Reading will always accompany the meals of the brothers. . . . Let there be complete silence. No whispering, no speaking – only the reader's voice should be heard there.

Saint Benedict, *The Rule of Saint Benedict*

Do you ever feel the presence of the divine as you eat? The ancient prayer practice of sacred reading (*lectio divina*) opens you to an interpersonal relationship with the divine. This is deep prayerful listening and receptiveness.

Set your intention to meet the divine. Next, choose a short passage – three to four paragraphs – of scripture or poetry. Read aloud, slowly and softly, as if hearing it for the first time and as if it is offered especially for you. Reflect silently until a word or phrase speaks to you. Say this word softly.

Now, recite the passage again. This time, listen for a deeper meaning of your chosen word or phrase. Now, say "I hear . . ." or "I see . . ." whatever it is that is being shared with you.

The third reading leads you into understanding what the divine communicates to you. This can be experienced as what you need to do or change. After reading and reflecting, begin by saying, "I believe God (the divine) wants me to . . ."

◆

Try sacred reading before, during, or after your meal.

Community

If you shift your focus from yourself to others,
extend your concern to others . . . then this will
have the immediate effect of opening up your life
and helping you to reach out.

DALAI LAMA, *Transforming the Mind*

DO YOU NOTICE HUNGRY AND UNDERNOURISHED people in your community? Do you ever see them on TV? Do you ever get approached during holidays and asked to make donations for the hungry? The next time this happens, pay attention to how it makes you feel about your own emotional issues around food.

Sometimes, the problem of hunger – in the world and our own community – seems so overwhelming that the impulse may be to ignore or deny it. But sometimes, facing the pain of others can help you deal with and recognize your own emotional pain.

Do you have spiritual heroes or people you admire for how they help or feed others? There is only one thing that separates you from them: your next action. It is that simple for you to reach out. And as you feed the hunger of others, watch how your own emotional hunger changes.

✦

Reflect on how turning to your
community can heal your own emotional
pain and food issue.

Departure

Over the winter glaciers,
I see the summer glow,
And through the wild-piled snowdrift
The warm rose buds below.

RALPH WALDO EMERSON

DO YOU BRING HARMONY AND BALANCE TO YOUR body after eating? Do you listen to your body closely? Or do you continue to eat and nibble even though you are no longer hungry? In the winter, a farmer must wait until the thaw before knowing what seeds to plant. For you, the "thaw" must be felt in your body.

When you have finished eating you can tune in to what your body needs at this moment – even if your mind thinks differently. Begin by sitting in a chair and taking a mindful breath.

As you begin to scan your body, place your attention on your feet. Feel how they touch the floor. Do they feel bloated, fatigued, tense, or at ease? Continue to scan your calves, thighs, hips, intestines, stomach, heart, lungs, torso, hands, arms, shoulders, neck, face, and skull.

Let this experience inform you about how the foods you eat are working and what your body needs right now – rest or exercise.

◆

Listen to your body after mealtime
for better harmony.

Entry

My wife is a light eater. As soon as it's light,
she starts to eat.

HENNY YOUNGMAN, COMEDIAN

DO YOU EAT AT EVERY OPPORTUNITY? ARE YOU always on the hunt for more food? Is the impulse to eat triggered just by seeing an advertisement or a restaurant? If this is a persistent habit for you, then you can take positive steps to bring balance and harmony into the coming year.

The first step in understanding your food triggers is to become more aware of them. Here are a few common ones: You worked hard and deserve a reward; you feel tired and need an energy boost; you feel disappointed about something and you want to elevate your mood; you are bored and want something to do; you are stressed and want to soothe yourself.

Do any of these triggers sound or feel familiar? In you journal, note the situations and the emotions that they trigger (sadness, anger, boredom, etc.), as well as your resulting eating behavior.

◆

Look for themes and emotions around
compulsive eating.

Choices

So much of our selves went into raising this crop. . . . It is a harvest we could never have foreseen or obtained all on our own. It is the brilliant product of our co-creation with God.

MARY MANIN MORRISSEY, MINISTER

AS YOUR CYCLE OF EXPLORING FOOD COMES TO a close, it is appropriate that the last theme is choices. *Meal by Meal*, choice by choice, you shape your well-being. You are not alone in this, of course. You have put a lot of effort into "raising this crop" that you are still harvesting and cocreating each moment.

Each moment brings new choices. No matter how many times you have chosen path A in the past year, you can choose path B or C or D in this next moment and in the New Year. In fact, you are probably already more skillful in your choices than you imagine.

As I write this final meditation, I choose to eat a green, tart, sweet Granny Smith apple. This is my year-end celebration apple. Each crunchy bite sprays my taste buds with juice. Chewing, chewing, the flesh mashes down with jaw-bending chomp-a-chomp-a-chomp until only the firm skin remains between my teeth and the sweetness evaporates with a swallow. I watch as the core turns yellow and the small seeds, dark brown, wait for a new season.

◆

With mindfulness may your New Year bring healthy, joyful choices and awareness – of food, emotion, relationships!

Author's Note

WRITING *Meal By Meal* WAS A WONDERFUL EXPERIENCE. Personally, it enabled me to bring mindfulness to readers in daily, "bite-sized" pieces. And while writing a book is satisfying, it completes only half the circle of what it means to bring a work like this (or any work) into the world. The other half is hearing from you and learning your experiences with these meditations. Would you share some of your experiences with me? On the one hand, this could be useful as feedback for my future work. On another level, it affirms the web of connection by which all our stories are interwoven.

I invite you to contact me through my web site:
www.mindfulpractices.com
and I will do my best to reply to each e-mail that
has "Meal-by-Meal Experience" in the subject line.

All Blessings and Peace,
Donald Altman